HI-TECH BABIES

Alternative Reproductive Technologies

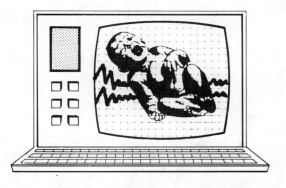

Gary E. McCuen

IDEAS IN CONFLICT SERIES

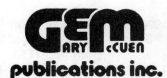

publications inc.

502 Second Street
Hudson, Wisconsin 54016
Phone (715) 386-7113

Illustration & photo credits

Brookins 48, Robert Gorrell 113, Steve Kelly 124, Craig MacIntosh 97, Office of Technology Assessment 26, 32, 45, 62, 74, 90, 110, 146, Steve Sack 137, William Sanders 131, David Seavey 55, 68, 80, 85, 103, 143, Stahler 18, Signe Wilkinson 39. Cover illustration by Ron Swanson.

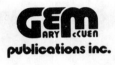

©1990 by Gary E. McCuen Publications, Inc. 502 Second Street, Hudson, Wisconsin 54016 (715) 386-7113 International Standard Book Number 0-86596-077-1 Printed in the United States of America

CONTENTS

CHAPTER 4   SURROGATE MOTHERS

CHAPTER 5 NEW CONCEPTIONS AND
GOVERNMENT REGULATION

REASONING SKILL DEVELOPMENT

These activities may be used as individualized study guides for students in libraries and resource centers or as discussion catalysts in small group and classroom discussions.

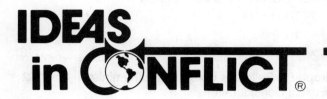

IDEAS in CONFLICT ®

This series features ideas in conflict on political, social and moral issues. It presents counterpoints, debates, opinions, commentary and analysis for use in libraries and classrooms. Each title in the series uses one or more of the following basic elements:

Introductions that present an issue overview giving historic background and/or a description of the controversy.

Counterpoints and debates carefully chosen from publications, books, and position papers on the political right and left to help librarians and teachers respond to requests that treatment of public issues be fair and balanced.

Symposiums and forums that go beyond debates that can polarize and oversimplify. These present commentary from across the political spectrum that reflect how complex issues attract many shades of opinion.

A global emphasis with foreign perspectives and surveys on various moral questions and political issues that will help readers to place subject matter in a less culture-bound and ethno-centric frame of reference. In an ever shrinking and interdependent world, understanding and cooperation are essential. Many issues are global in nature and can be effectively dealt with only by common efforts and international understanding.

Reasoning skill study guides and discussion activities provide ready made tools for helping with critical reading and evaluation of content. The guides and activities deal with one or more of the following:

RECOGNIZING AUTHOR'S POINT OF VIEW

INTERPRETING EDITORIAL CARTOONS

VALUES IN CONFLICT

WHAT IS EDITORIAL BIAS?

6

WHAT IS SEX BIAS?
WHAT IS POLITICAL BIAS?
WHAT IS ETHNOCENTRIC BIAS?
WHAT IS RACE BIAS?
WHAT IS RELIGIOUS BIAS?

*From across **the political spectrum** varied sources are presented for research projects and classroom discussions. Diverse opinions in the series come from magazines, newspapers, syndicated columnists, books, political speeches, foreign nations, and position papers by corporations and non-profit institutions.*

About the Editor

Gary E. McCuen is an editor and publisher of anthologies for public libraries and curriculum materials for schools. Over the past 19 years his publications of over 200 titles have specialized in social, moral and political conflict. They include books, pamphlets, cassettes, tabloids, filmstrips and simulation games, many of them designed from his curriculums during 11 years of teaching junior and senior high school social studies. At present he is the editor and publisher of the *Ideas in Conflict* series and the *Editorial Forum* series.

CHAPTER 1

NEW REPRODUCTIVE TECHNOLOGIES: AN OVERVIEW

1 NEW REPRODUCTIVE TECHNOLOGIES: AN OVERVIEW

FERTILITY AND INFERTILITY

Office of Technology Assessment

Excerpted from *Infertility: Medical and Social Choices,* Office of Technology
Assessment, May 1988, pp. 1-12.

How Big a Problem Is Infertility?

Infertility, generally defined as the inability of a couple to conceive after 12 months of intercourse without contraception, affects an estimated 2.4 million married couples (data from 1982) and an unknown number of would-be parents among unmarried couples and singles. It is an important personal and societal problem. . . .

Childlessness, or primary infertility, has increased and affects about 1.0 million couples. Secondary infertility (in which couples have at least one biological child) has decreased and affects about 1.4 million couples. Surgical sterilization has increased dramatically. Certain couples are more likely than others to be infertile: the incidence among blacks, for example, is 1.5 times higher than among whites.

It is noteworthy that not all infertile couples seek treatment. An estimated 51 percent of couples with primary infertility and 22 percent with secondary infertility seek treatment. . . .

Three factors most often contribute to infertility among women: problems in ovulation, blocked or scarred fallopian tubes, and endometriosis (the presence in the lower abdomen of tissue from the uterine lining). Infections with sexually transmitted diseases (STDs), principally chlamydia and gonorrhea, are an important cause of damaged fallopian tubes. Among men, most cases of infertility are a consequence of abnormal or too few sperm. For as many as one in five infertile couples, a cause is never found. . . .

Infertility resulting from sexually transmitted diseases — an estimated 20 percent of the cases in the United States — is the most preventable. In these instances, prevention of infertility equals prevention (and rapid and effective treatment) of sexually transmitted diseases. The risk of infertility increases with the number of times a person has chlamydia or gonorrhea, the duration and severity of each infection, and any delay in instituting treatment.

Effective public health initiatives aimed at preventing STDs and infertility include efforts in the following areas:

- health education of patients and public health professionals;
- disease definition, including long-term sequelae of STDs;
- optimal treatment and improved clinical service;
- partner tracing and patient counseling; and research, including the social, psychological, and biologic aspects of STDs. . . .

How Is Infertility Diagnosed and Treated?

Among infertile couples seeking treatment, 85 to 90 percent are treated with conventional medical and surgical therapy. Medical treatment ranges from instructing the couple in the relatively simple methods of pinpointing ovulation to more complex treatments involving ovulation induction with powerful fertility drugs and artificial insemination. Surgical treatments also span a wide spectrum of complexity. . . .

What Ethical Issues Are Involved?

A wide range of conflicting established moral viewpoints makes the development of public policy related to infertility difficult. Where there are pluralities of viewpoints and a lack of any single established moral approach, uniform solutions are questionable.

Recent years have seen the appearance of several ethical analyses of reproductive technologies, with most leading to pronouncements that a particular technology is either ethically acceptable or not. In 1987, for example, the Roman Catholic Church issued its *Instruction on Respect for Human Life in Its Origin and on the Dignity of Procreation*. The Church supported basic medical and surgical treatment for infertility but opposed nearly all other techniques for diagnosing and treating infertility.

Similar analyses examine at least six themes:

- **The right to reproduce.** Procreation is seen by most as a fundamental facet of being human. Differing views about the relative importance of procreation have spawned disagreement over how to balance a claim to reproduce against other needs. Critical unanswered questions are whether infertile couples have the right to use the gametes or bodies of others, and the right to financial assistance to obtain treatment they might not otherwise be able to afford.

- **The moral status of an embryo.** In vitro fertilization (IVF) and the ability to freeze embryos raise questions about appropriate treatment of embryos that are likely to be debated for some time to come. While some recognize embryos as full persons from the moment of fertilization, others claim embryos have no moral status whatsoever. Still others contend embryos have significant moral standing, although not equal to that of people. The unresolved debate about how to view and handle human embryos has impeded the growth of new knowledge about fertility, infertility, and contraception.

- **Bonding between parent and child.** Parent-child bonding is

11

important both to parents and to the developing personality of the child. Conception that involves the efforts of a third party may redefine parenthood. The use of reproductive technologies raises questions about the minimum requirements for bonding and the meaning of parent-child relationships—and what they ought to be.

- **Research with patients**. Infertile patients have a right to know when treatment is a proven medical therapy and when it amounts to an experimental trial. Further, because of their often intense effort to conceive, infertile patients are particularly vulnerable to abuses of the researcher-subject relationship.

- **Truth-telling and confidentiality.** The intimate nature of infertility diagnosis and treatment and the use of donor gametes complicates simple ethical imperatives to tell the truth and to hold personal information in confidence.

- **Responsibilities of one generation to another.** Parents, physicians, and researchers have a duty to refrain from using reproductive technologies in ways that might harm future generations.

Most religious traditions in the United States view necessary medical or surgical treatments for infertility as acceptable and hold them to be desirable. There is general acceptance of the morality of artificial insemination by husband, considerable hesitation about artificial insemination by donor, and even less support for artificial insemination of single women. Most religions support IVF or gamete intrafallopian transfer using the married couple's own sperm and eggs as long as no embryos are discarded. Surrogate motherhood is largely opposed in any form. . . .

What Does the Law Say?

The U.S. Constitution has been interpreted to preclude almost any kind of governmental effort to prevent competent individuals from marrying and exercising their innate fertility. Yet there is no explicit statement in the Constitution of either a right to procreate or a right to privacy. Court decisions do not clearly state whether such rights extend to a right to obtain medical services, to use donor gametes, to use a surrogate mother, or to pay for these three avenues of overcoming infertility. Nevertheless, any governmental effort to regulate or ban any aspect of noncoital reproduction is certain to be subjected to judicial scrutiny.

Issues likely to be before the courts in the coming years

include regulation of medical treatments using a couple's own gametes, restrictions on use of embryos not transferred, payment for undergoing medical procedures that carry some risk (e.g., ova donation), payment for embryos and their transfer, and the government's obligation to pay for or otherwise provide infertility services for poor people.

2 NEW REPRODUCTIVE TECHNOLOGIES: AN OVERVIEW

ARTIFICIAL HUMAN REPRODUCTION: PROS AND CONS

House Select Committee on Children, Youth, and Families

Excerpted from a minority report of the House Select Committee on Children, Youth, and Families, May 21, 1987.

In Vitro Fertilization (IVF)

Definition

A woman is put on hormonal therapy to stimulate egg production, then her eggs are harvested and fertilized with her husband's sperm (or from a sperm bank donor's) in the laboratory. Several of the fertilized eggs are returned to the uterus of the original donor or a surrogate mother. In vitro (Latin for "in glass"), once known as test-tube fertilization, is commonly recommended for women with some abnormality or blockage in the fallopian tubes.

Four Key Methods:

(1) The wife's egg can be fertilized by the husband's sperm in the petri dish and implanted in the wife (2 parents);

(2) Another woman's egg can be fertilized by the husband's sperm in the petri dish and implanted in the wife (3 parents);

(3) Another woman's egg can be fertilized by another man's sperm in the petri dish and implanted in the wife (4 parents);

(4) Another woman's egg can be fertilized by another man's sperm in the petri dish and implanted in yet another woman, then raised by the family that originally desired child (5 parents).

Other Key Definitions

Embryo: The infant during the 2nd through 8th week after fertilization.

Infertility: The inability among men to fertilize eggs is usually due to low sperm count or weak sperm; the inability of women's eggs to become fertilized is most often due to tubal blockage.

Cryopreservation: A method of freezing for later use embryos that remain after an initial implantation attempt (there are many such clinics throughout the country, including Fairfax County). Embryos or sperm are frozen at a temperature of approximately -200^0 C in liquid nitrogen; when needed they are thawed slowly and transferred into a recipient's uterus.

Laparoscopy: A telescope-like instrument is inserted through a small incision in the patient's abdomen, which enables doctors to see the ova; then a long, thin needle is inserted through a second incision, and ova with surrounding fluid are carefully removed and placed in a laboratory dish (petri dish). (Note: In some cases this does not work and several other new technologies have been developed for these exceptions.)

Test-tube baby: A baby born through in vitro fertilization.

Embryo replacement: When the embryo is returned to the donor.

Embryo transfer: When the embryo is implanted into a recipient other than the donor of the ovum (i.e., egg). . . .

Key Issues of In Vitro Fertilization

(1) *Should the procedure be performed on humans?*

Yes

Affords childless couples the chance to bear children, which they may not otherwise have.

Biomedical science is constantly teaching us new facts about ourselves, and biomedical technology is providing us as persons with new capacities to control our environments and to make genetically-transmissible changes in ourselves.

Dr. Leroy Walters: The nature of the technology itself is less important than the social and political uses to which the technology is put. (His argument is that the debate should not be the technology but how some propose to use it.)

Professor Joseph Fletcher: He welcomes the new and artificial modes of reproduction as a much-needed alternative to what he calls the traditional coital-gestational method. He argues that only by employing such new methods will we be able to "end reproductive roulette" and begin to reduce our overwhelming load of genetic defects.

A possible comprehensive national program might work by comparing cards from various tests when marriage licenses are applied for. The couple could unite anyway but on the condition that Denmark makes, that sterilization is done for one or both of them. And they could still have children by medical and donor assistance, bypassing their own faulty fertility. (Joseph Fletcher)

No

Replaces conception that originates from a natural intercourse with that of an unnatural origin, conception in a dish outside the body.

Professor Paul Ramsey: "We shall have to assess in vitro fertilization as a long step toward Hatcheries; that is extracorporeal gestation, and the introduction of unlimited genetic changes into human germinal material while it is cultured by the Conditioners and Predestinators of the future."

Vatican document titled "Instruction on Respect for Human Life in Its Origin and on the Dignity of Procreation": In vitro

16

fertilization between husband and wife is unacceptable because "even if it is considered in the context of 'de facto' existing sexual relations, the generation of the human person is objectively deprived of its proper perfection: namely, that of being the result and fruit of a conjugal act."

Catholic theologian Michael Novak: The document's main thrust "is to defend a human right never before articulated in such detail and clarity: the human right of a child to be born to two married persons through the mutual gift of their bodily and personal love for one another."

Lutheran theologian Richard John Neuhaus: "I don't think it's [the Vatican document] the definite word, but it's a marvelously good starting point for discussion. . . it seems to be a limited definition of the act of love but one is challenged to ask, if you expand the act of love to separate love from the act of procreation, then where do you draw the line? It has raised a challenge to all of us to be more precise."

(2) What legal status should an embryo have? Should it have all the legal rights of a human being?

This is especially complicated in view of freezing of embryos for indefinite periods of time.

What provision should be made for embryos in the case where the donors separate or die?

If the donors die, as they did in an Australian plane crash in 1983, and if the embryo is implanted and later delivered, what are the inheritance rights of the child?

(3) Whose child is it?

In 1954 in the Illinois case *Doornbos v. Doornbos*, the court held that even if her husband had consented, a woman who underwent artificial insemination by donor was guilty of adultery. More recent court rulings hold that if a married woman is artificially inseminated with the consent of her husband, the child is the legal child of that couple.

Many state statutes specifically provide that a man is not the legal father if he furnishes sperm for artificial insemination of a woman who is not his wife.

(4) Independence for Women

Jane Mattes, a psychotherapist, founded Single Mothers by Choice. "Relationships now are disposable. People split. Being a parent is a place to work out intimacy where your partner can't leave."

Women no longer have to settle on a man just because time is

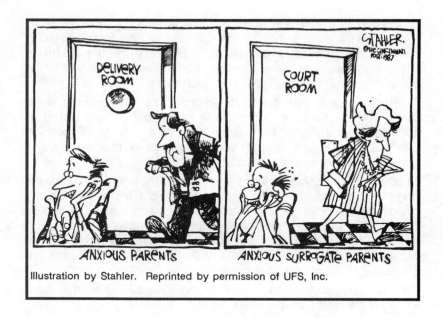

DELIVERY ROOM

COURT ROOM

STAHLER.
©THE CINCINNATI POST·1987

ANXIOUS PARENTS

ANXIOUS SURROGATE PARENTS

Illustration by Stahler. Reprinted by permission of UFS, Inc.

running out on their biological clock and single men can seek a surrogate mother if they do not want the entanglements of a wife. (*Life* magazine cover story; June, 1987)

(5) Who should be responsible for the costs of IVF?

Many researchers believe that the federal government, which funds the major portion of all biomedical research in the U.S., should support IVF research.

"Just as there are people who would like to buy a fine car, and have to settle for something else, so there are people who cannot afford this."—Dr. Howard Jones, Eastern Medical School in Norfolk, Virginia.

Artificial Insemination

Definition

Sperm from an anonymous donor provides a common solution for a male infertility problem. Increasingly, sperm banks are freezing supplies so that, for instance, a couple who want more than one child can go back several years later for a second insemination from the same donor, making their children true siblings.

Key Facts

Thousands of births (3,576 in 1977) by this method.

95 percent in one survey were because of male infertility (*New*

England Journal of Medicine, "Current Practice of Artificial Insemination by Donor in the United States," March 15, 1979).

40 percent of the doctors surveyed have provided this service for reasons other than male sterility however, including those husbands who feared transmitting a genetic disease. *(NEJ of Medicine).*

10 percent of the doctors in this 1977 survey inseminated single women *(NEJ of Medicine).*

62 percent of doctors who selected their own donors for patients used medical students or hospital residents *(NEJ of Medicine).*

Most doctors attempted to match at least hair color, skin color, eye color and height; more than half also considered religious or ethnic background and blood types. *(NEJ of Medicine).*

Most doctors who kept track of this information (and fewer doctors answered this question than any other) had never used a donor for more than 6 pregnancies. Approximately 6 percent had used donors for 15 or more pregnancies. *(NEJ of Medicine).*

Special Problem with This Method of Birth

Using a single donor for many recipients may result in inadvertent consanguinity or inbreeding. This complication could occur if two people mated who unknowingly shared the same genetic father or if a recipient was inseminated with the semen of a relative. Either may occur accidentally, since the identity of the semen donor is almost always concealed.

Confidentiality of donors also raises problems relating to possible future questions regarding adoption, genetic counseling, psychologic needs, and other such questions.

Pro

"'Once upon a time there was a man and a woman. They met, fell in love and married. And very soon they decided to have a family. They made love, and within a year, their first child was born. That one was very soon followed by others. And they lived happily ever after.' THIS IS A FAIRY TALE. For millions of people in America in 1987, it is as patently fantastic as Sleeping Beauty."—*Life* magazine cover story, June, 1987

"Clergy who have talked often of the family as the linchpin of life now say that they want to restrict how families can be created." *Life,* 1987

Procreation is separated from sexual intercourse but in some cases only when the couple has determined that sexual intercourse does not lead to procreation in any case. In these cases, some see the physician functioning as a kind of early midwife, helping the couple with the beginnings of the pregnancy rather than with the delivery of a fully developed fetus.

Con

From "Instruction on Respect for Human Life in Its Origin and on the Dignity of Procreation":

"The fidelity of the spouses in the unity of marriage involves reciprocal respect of their right to become a father and a mother only through each other."

"Heterologous artificial fertilization is contrary to the unity of marriage, to the dignity of the spouses, to the vocation proper to parents, and to the child's right to be conceived and brought into the world in marriage and from marriage."

"The fertilization of a married woman with the sperm of a donor different from her husband and fertilization with the husband's sperm of an ovum not coming from his wife are morally illicit. Furthermore, the artificial fertilization of a woman who is unmarried or a widow, whoever the donor may be, cannot be morally justified."

"Homologous artificial fertilization, in seeking a procreation which is not fruit of a specific act of conjugal union, objectively effects an analogous separation between the goods and the meanings of marriage."

"Masturbation, through which the sperm is normally obtained, is another sign of this dissociation: Even when it is done for the purpose of procreation the act remains deprived of its unitive meaning: 'It lacks the sexual relationship called for by the moral order, namely the relationship which realizes the full sense of mutual self-giving and human procreation in the context of true love.'"

Surrogate Motherhood

Definition

A surrogate motherhood arrangement generally involves a couple that is infertile or otherwise unable or unwilling to bear a child, and a woman, contracted by the couple to bear the child for them.

In the process, a woman, or surrogate, is impregnated by the semen of a man who is not her husband and agrees to turn over the child born as a result of that action to the child's father and his wife. Although circumstances of particular cases can vary, the parties generally sign a contract setting out their various rights and responsibilities, under which the surrogate mother agrees to relinquish all rights to the child after birth, in exchange for a fee (typically $10,000) and payment of all legal and medical expenses. The father's wife is not usually party to this contract, to avoid possible violation and prohibitions against "baby selling," but goes on to legally adopt the child as her own, after her husband's paternity has been established. Following this action, unless otherwise provided by contract, the surrogate mother has no legal right to further contact with the child.

Other types of surrogate mothering arrangements exist, such as those between a surrogate and a single male, an unmarried couple or a single woman who can not or will not carry the child and does not want the burden of a spouse. For the most part, however, surrogate arrangements involve a couple and a woman to act as a surrogate.

The use of the term "surrogate" for a woman who is the genetic and gestational mother of a child appears a misnomer to those who feel that the adoptive mother is actually the surrogate for the biologic mother, who has given up her child.

Specifics of the Process and Contracting Procedure

When the wife has been determined to be infertile (or has problems that preclude pregnancy) and generally after other methods of fertilization have been exhausted, the couple may seek legal and medical advice for an arrangement with a surrogate mother. A lawyer is charged with finding a surrogate and preparing the legal documents for the procedure. Generally, these documents arrange payment of the surrogate and clarify that in return she must turn over the child and all further responsibility and legal right to the child. It further provides that the father has the right to demand that the mother undergo amniocentesis to determine if the fetus is deformed, and can insist that the mother have an abortion based on the results of the test. While financial arrangements may vary, most set out a schedule of payments should the mother miscarry or give birth to a stillborn child, in addition to the payment of all medical and legal expenses. The father is usually thought obligated to accept a physically or mentally deformed child, although this may not be specifically spelled out in the contract.

After a series of tests, the surrogate mother is artificially inseminated with the semen of the contracting husband. By contract, the mother is bound not to have sex with anyone during this process until her pregnancy is confirmed. Her actions, eating and drinking habits, and other aspects of her personal life are controlled by the contract and the father may disclaim responsibility or default on the contract subject to the mother's observance of the contractual obligations.

After the birth of the child and the determination of its health, the mother has a certain period (depending on the contract and the state law) in which she may reconsider surrendering the child. Once she decides to relinquish responsibility for the infant and the father's paternity is established, the process of adoption by the father's wife may take place, thus the couple takes the child as their own. . . .

Pro

"Collaborative reproduction allows some persons who might otherwise remain childless to produce healthy children."

"For couples exhausted and frustrated by these efforts [to adopt a child] the surrogate arrangement seems a godsend."

"While this price tag [$20,000 to $25,000] makes the surrogate contract a consumption item for the middle classes, it is not unjust to poor couples for it does not leave them worse off than they were."

"If you estimate 600 to date, the percentage of problems is very, very small. This is the last alternative for many people. They have already gone through surgery, in vitro fertilization, an adoption attempt. They know there are not enough adoptable babies. They feel very lucky that there is one more alternative."

"For the child, the use of a surrogate mother gives him or her an opportunity that would not otherwise be available: the opportunity to exist. Furthermore, the child would be reared by a couple who so wanted him or her that they were willing to participate in a novel process with potential legal and other risks."

Con

"Surrogate motherhood is partly like indentured servitude and partly like prostitution. Like prostitution, it makes one of the most intimate acts a commercial, and therefore, impersonal, transaction. Like indentured servitude, it permits an individual to sell, not just the fruits of his labor, but his personal autonomy."

"In exalting promiscuity to the level of monogamy, and reducing motherhood to a 'service,' we pander to the weakest side of our natures and punish what is best in us."

"However, its [surrogate mothering's] deliberate separation of genetic, gestational, and social parentage is troublesome. . .

there is a risk of confusing family lineage and personal identity. In addition, the techniques intentionally manipulate a natural process that many persons want free of technical intervention."

"Surrogate mother arrangements are designed to separate in the mind of the surrogate mother the decision to create a child from the decision to have and raise that child. The cause of this dissociation is some other benefit that she will receive, most often money. In other words, her desire to create a child is born of some motive other than the desire to become a parent. This separation of the decision to create a child from the decision to parent it is ethically suspect. The child is conceived not because he is wanted by his biological mother, but because he can be useful to someone else. He is conceived in order to be given away."

Alternative Methods of Surrogacy

Host womb surrogacy

It is now possible to fertilize an egg outside of the body through in vitro fertilization, and use the resultant embryo to impregnate a surrogate mother if the biological mother for some reason cannot carry a child. Also, embryo transplants may in time make it possible for women with histories of early miscarriages to become pregnant, after which the embryo is moved to the womb of another woman who carries and gives birth to the child.

The world's first 'host womb' baby (the mother's egg was fertilized in vitro by the father's sperm and implanted into the womb of a third woman) recently turned one year old. . . .

Should research on human embryos be permitted?

Proponents: Research on embryos should be allowed in order to gain knowledge which could be aimed, not only at improving the success rate of in vitro fertilization, but also at increasing researcher's understanding about the early stages of human development (Irene Stith-Coleman, Analyst in Life Sciences, Science Policy Research Division, Congressional Research Service, April 12, 1985).

Opponents: It would be unethical to experiment on human embryos because, to do so, is to tamper with human life, which is viewed as sacred. Opponents also fear that scientists may potentially use the knowledge obtained from research on human embryos to produce people with selective physical and mental characteristics (Irene Stith-Coleman, Analyst in Life Sciences, Science Policy Research Division, Congressional Research Service, April 12, 1985). . . .

Amniocentesis and Ultrasound

Prenatal diagnosis of the baby's expected condition.

Pro

It is claimed that some children are now born healthy because doctors can judge when and how to deliver and arrange for pediatric surgeons to be present in the delivery room, ready to perform immediate procedures.

Con

It is claimed that the methods are primarily used to identify unwanted children so that they can be aborted.

"The most advanced machines now provide images good enough that pregnant women often stare in amazed delight at the screen, waving and talking to their fetuses as they roll and kick before their eyes. The machine, however, requires an educated, practiced eye to sort out the blurred gray shapes and understand what they mean."—from *Los Angeles Times* article by Barry Siegel.

"He knew his burden. To conclude whether a thumbnail-size heart was normal probably would decide the fetus' fate and affect the parents in unknown ways. If someone is going to terminate a pregnancy based on my diagnosis, he told himself, I'm going to be sure. But then he thought: We're not perfect. We're not God." "'I feel uncomfortable to a degree,' he said slowly, choosing each word with care. 'But not so uncomfortable as to change what I do here. . . There is a recognition that we aren't perfect, that our attempts to improve people's lives do a fair amount of good and also cause problems.'"—*LA Times*

"A couple's firstborn suffered from a particular type of mental retardation and organ malformation that was marked physically by small dysplastic fingernails. During the second pregnancy, the doctors were asked to examine the fetus.

"It was, as always, a judgment call. They had limited experience then, and the few other cases they had seen had been during varying points of gestation. Still, they both agree that it seemed like the fingernails were malformed. The fetus looked afflicted. The family decided to terminate. Afterward, the doctor studied the tiny abortus. Try as he might, he could not convince himself that the fingernails were abnormal. Nor could the other doctors."—*LA Times*

THE GENIUS SPERM BANK: POINTS AND COUNTERPOINTS

This activity may be used as an individualized study guide for students in libraries and resource centers or as a discussion catalyst in small group and classroom discussions.

The Point

In Escondido, California, a unique and potentially valuable experiment has been set up by Robert Clark Graham, a proponent of selective breeding. In this remarkable experiment, he has made frozen sperm from his genius sperm bank available to interested infertile couples. At least 55 children have come into the world via artificial insemination from Robert Clark Graham's sperm bank. Only sperm from superior people (IQ above 130), who have no history of genetic problems or disease, are selected. Robert Clark Graham is not in it for the money. A modest fee of $10 per sperm shipment and $50 for paperwork has been his typical charge. He is simply trying to make couples happy and help the world produce gifted children who can offer leadership to help solve the most serious global problems.

The Counterpoint

The theory that superior people should be encouraged to reproduce while those less capable should be prohibited, penalized, or discouraged from having children, is a dangerous social problem. This notion of eugenics still has followers today. One example is the sperm bank in Escondido, California. This sordid theory of eugenics in America's recent past led to the sterilization of thousands of "unfit" mentally retarded and feeble-minded people. The term "unfit" was highly subjective and also applied to alcoholics, sexual deviants, and those suffering from criminal behavior. Notions of eugenics have been used to justify emigration quotas on racial grounds, euthanasia,

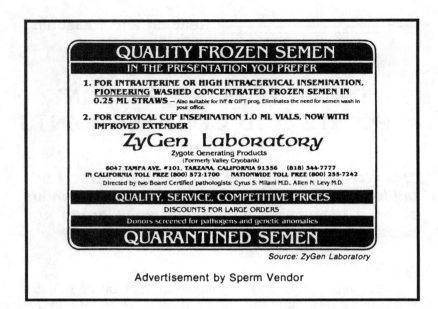
and genocide against Jews and political prisoners in Nazi Germany.

Guidelines

1. Examine the counterpoints.

2. Which argument do you agree with more and why?

3. Social issues are usually complex, but often problems become oversimplified in political debates and discussions. Usually a polarized version of social conflict does not adequately represent the diversity of views that surround social conflicts. Examine the counterpoints. Then write down possible interpretations of the issue other than the two arguments stated in the counterpoints.

CHAPTER 2

MOVING TOWARD EUGENICS?

MOVING TOWARD EUGENICS?

THE SEARCH FOR A
PERFECT CHILD

Jerry E. Bishop and Michael Waldholz

*Jerry E. Bishop and Michael Waldholz cover science and medicine
for* The Wall Street Journal.

Points to Consider:

1. What is the Michael Reese Medical Center? Where is it lo-
   cated? What did researchers there discover?

2. Describe the new gene-identification technology. What issues has it raised?

3. Define the term "eugenics."

4. How should our society deal with genetic tampering?

History indicates that any time it becomes possible to alter a human trait, the definitions of "health" and "disease" suddenly change.

Within the first few hours after conception a phenomenon takes place in the one-cell human embryo that has awed scientists and philosophers for more than a century. The genes of the mother, carried by the ovum, and the genes of the father, carried by the sperm, pair up. At that moment, when the pairing is completed, the genetic fate of the person-to-be is sealed. The sex, color of eyes and hair, the height, blood type, fingerprints, shoe size—indeed, all physical and chemical characteristics—are irrevocably determined.

Suppose, then, one could look into this embryo when division has proceeded to four or eight microscopic cells. If a deleterious or undesirable combination of genes is discovered, the cells could be discarded and a second conception initiated in hope of achieving a more desirable genetic combination.

Anyone thinking such technology lies in the distant future should take note of research at Michael Reese Medical Center in Chicago, which offers a test-tube fertilization service to infertile women. Using microscopic human test-tube embryos that were about to be discarded because they were developing abnormally, researchers there were able to detect a number of genes in the embryos when they had advanced only to the four-cell stage.

Far-Reaching Implications

"Preliminary studies with human embryos rejected for implantation suggest that in the future it may be possible to monitor high-risk pregnancies by embryonic biopsy, transferring [to the woman] only those [embryos] determined to be genetically unaffected and thereby eliminating the need for prenatal testing," the Chicago scientists said recently in the *American Journal of Human Genetics.*

The experiment only hints at the more far-reaching implications of an explosive new technology that is being pursued by the world's biological laboratories. This technology involves the ability to locate and isolate individual genes in human cells. As the articles reported, this new gene-identification technology already is leading to the first prenatal tests for such genetic disorders as muscular dystrophy, cystic fibrosis, hemophilia and Huntington's disease.

29

The New Technology

In the near future, perhaps a few years or even months, the new technology will enable doctors and parents to test new-born infants or unborn fetuses for scores of different genes, some of which cause heredity diseases and some of which only predispose the developing fetus to diseases in the future. The genes that predispose a person to heart disease in middle age are now being uncovered, for example. And the search is on for genes that predispose one to cancer, arthritis, ulcers, depression, schizophrenia, alcoholism and even criminal behavior.

This new technology raises immediate social and ethical problems, ranging from whether abortions should be permitted for a disease that won't manifest itself until adulthood to the use of genetic screening by employers, insurers or even the government to deny a person a job or a promotion or to determine his or her niche in society.

But such experiments as those at Michael Reese hint at an issue that so far hasn't been raised by either the scientists or the sociologists. This is the possibility that the new technology will lead, perhaps inadvertently, to a eugenics* program.

---

*Editor's note: According to the *American Heritage Dictionary*, eugenics is "the study of hereditary improvement, especially of human improvement by genetic control."

A Eugenics Program?

The broadening use of prenatal diagnoses by the current generation of "baby-boomers" suggests that young couples already are going to considerable lengths to ensure the birth of a near-perfect child. Tens of thousands of women, many in their early 30s, currently are undergoing prenatal testing at 16 weeks of pregnancy to avoid the birth of a child with any of a number of genetic defects such as mental retardation. Genetic counselors say they occasionally encounter couples who, whatever their stated reasons, are seeking a prenatal test solely to determine the sex of the fetus and who, presumably, would have an abortion should the fetus be, say, a male instead of the desired female.

The current experiments suggest it soon will be technically possible for a young couple, in their desire to have an unblemished child, to have several of the woman's ova fertilized in the test tube with the husband's sperm producing several embryos with different genetic combinations. The embryo with the most desirable genetic traits could be selected for implanting in the woman to produce a pregnancy. This would avoid the risks of an abortion at 16 weeks to 18 weeks of pregnancy and thus be far safer. The discarding of only four microscopic cells in the test tube also may be more acceptable to those who may be uneasy about the morality of abortion.

Altering Human Traits

The more worrisome question isn't whether young couples will resort to this technique but what genetic traits they will select for their offspring. Scientists working with the new genetic technology say it's unthinkable that pregnancy and births would be prevented on grounds that the person-to-be might develop severe heart disease at age 25 or suffer the agony of depression in adulthood or might have criminal tendencies. They say their research is aimed at understanding disease and developing new treatments and cures, not at eugenics.

Yet history indicates that any time it becomes possible to alter a human trait, the definitions of "health" and "disease" suddenly change. A current example is short stature. In the past, dwarfs might have been considered unlucky but not necessarily diseased, while those who were below average in height were merely considered short.

The discovery of a hormone that controls growth has changed this definition. As a result, scores of children are currently being treated with human growth hormone—produced incidentally by

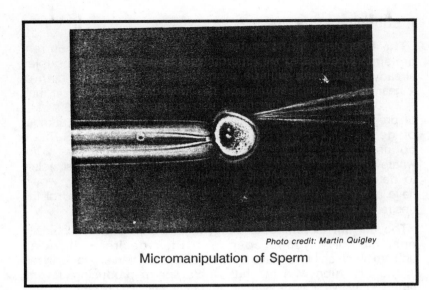

Micromanipulation of Sperm

genetic engineering techniques—for shortness. The gene for growth hormone has been isolated, and it soon may be possible to detect it in the fetus—or the test-tube embryo. Other substances that control growth and stature, and the genes that produce them, are certain to be discovered. Young couples in the future could very well have the choice of birthing a child who will grow to five feet or even six feet in height.

Genes That Govern Intelligence

Another choice that is likely to be available deals with intelligence. An indication of how close scientists are to uncovering at least some of the genes that govern intelligence comes from current research on a condition known as the fragile X chromosome. A half-dozen years ago it was discovered that a large portion of the mentally retarded males in institutions possessed an X chromosome that tended to break at the tip when grown in the test tube. An unusual aspect of these men with a fragile X chromosome was that, unlike other mentally retarded persons, they appeared to suffer few other physical or physiological defects. This suggested that the genes lying near the tip of the X chromosome may be intimately involved in mental development, and that the mental retardation of these men wasn't the secondary consequence of some gross physiological defect.

A prenatal test to detect the fragile X chromosome was

developed almost immediately, but wasn't used. It wasn't known if the fragile chromosome leads inevitably to mental retardation; if it doesn't, the use of the prenatal test might lead to abortions of fetuses that would have been normal.

Since then, a major scientific effort has determined that the fragile X chromosome is present in non-retarded persons. Some boys with the defect are autistic, some only mildly so. Other boys are hyperactive and many are slow learners. Among girls who have one normal X chromosome to partially offset the effects of their fragile X chromosome, only a few are severely retarded. Other girls with the defect are on the borderline between retarded and normal. And there are both boys and girls with the defect who seem normal.

These discoveries are leading, in turn, to an intensive effort to identify individual genes at the site where the fragile X chromosome tended to break. Identifying the genes should allow scientists to distinguish among fetuses those that would be retarded, those that would be autistic, those that would be slow learners and those that would be normal.

The Danger of Too Many Choices

This research, of course, could lead to new treatments or cures for mental short-comings due to the fragile X chromosome. But one of the implications is quite clear: some would-be parents within the near future would be presented with the choice of whether or not to bear a child whose defect or "disease" will be a learning disability or a likelihood of failing in school and requiring special education. Given the rapid progress in genetic research, it's likely that in future generations the choice won't be limited just to those families carrying the fragile X chromosome. Soon scientists will be able to identify genes that control various aspects of intelligence in any embryo. And given the desire for the perfect child that even the present generation seems to have, there seems to be little doubt about how prospective parents will deal with these choices.

There is little need to dwell on what a totalitarian society might attempt to do with this new ability to select human genetic traits. The Nazi attempt at a government-directed eugenics program, as crack-pot as it was, is lesson enough.

But even in democratic societies there will likely be demands that such genetic tampering be taken out of the hands of individuals whose decisions might be subject to whim or fashion or whose concepts of what traits are desirable and what are undesirable may differ from the majority. There also will be concern that human interference on a large scale with natural selection of genetic traits could endanger the species over the long run. Government regulation seems inevitable. Legislation setting criteria of, say, height and I.Q. scores for genetic selection may not be out of the question.

MOVING TOWARD EUGENICS?

DESIGNING OUR DESCENDANTS: ON THE THRESHOLD OF AN IMMENSE ABYSS

Catherine Maentanis

Catherine Maentanis wrote the following article in her capacity as a contributing writer to Liberty Report, *a monthly publication of the Moral Majority, Inc.*

Points to Consider:

1. Why did the nurse in New York resign from her position at an obstetric ward?

2. Who is Dr. J. C. Willke? What reasons does he offer to explain society's cheapened view of human life?

3. Who is Bernard Nathanson? What warning does he offer in regard to laboratory experimentation?

4. What will happen if the American people choose not to protest genetic manipulation?

Catherine Maentanis, "In-Vitro Fertilization: Masking the Nature of Killing the Unborn Child," *Liberty Report*, June 1988, p. 19.

Lacking any type of legal and moral restraints, the future holds a frightening picture as the fields of genetic engineering and in vitro fertilization develop and the laboratory becomes a breeding ground for designing America's descendants.

When the first "test tube" baby was born in July 1978, the world stood in awe. Modern science had scaled a barrier once thought insurmountable.

Supporters hailed the accomplishment as a miraculous advancement for modern technology.

Lack of Ethical Code

Critics warned that scientific inquiry would stop at nothing, especially when it's not restrained by an ethical code upholding the sanctity of human life.

As doctors and researchers began to indulge in self-worship and to revere the laboratories they worked in, pro-life advocates cried out in protest.

Small Regard for Human Life

One such protester was a nurse in a New York hospital who resigned from her position at an obstetric ward after finding herself an accomplice to murder.

Active in in vitro fertilization because she thought it was the new wave of science's future, the young woman soon realized that specialists in this field had small regard for human life and considered the unborn child nothing more than a laboratory guinea pig.

The nurse who, for legal purposes, wishes to be unnamed, described one particular case in which a woman, who had been receiving fertility drugs, became pregnant with seven babies (or fertilized embryos as doctors prefer to call them).

Terminating Babies

She said the doctor told the woman that she and the babies might not live through the pregnancy. The doctor's solution was to terminate five of the babies since the mother wanted only two children anyway. At the time the woman and her doctor chose to terminate the five babies, she was six months pregnant.

The doctor inserted a needle through the mother's abdominal wall into her uterus. Using ultrasonic guidance, he inserted the needle into the heart of each of the tiny babies and injected potassium chloride—a compound that adversely affects the heart. At the term of the woman's pregnancy, she delivered healthy twins with the remaining five babies dead.

Deep Grief

"At that point I felt like the assistant of Dr. Joseph Mengele" (a German Nazi physician who experimented with infant brain tissue), the nurse mourned.

Afterwards, she was continually depressed, feeling deep grief because she had assisted in five deaths. Nursing had been her entire life and she always assisted in sustaining life. This experience had placed her in a position where she helped kill.

"Pregnancy Reduction"

Dr. J. C. Willke, president of the National Right to Life, says this procedure is called "pregnancy reduction" to mask the nature of the practice.

Willke says that such semantics are consistently used to make the practice of murdering innocent unborn babies more palatable to the American people. But, as he points out, regardless of the words used, all experimentation with in vitro fertilization, embryo transfer, freezing and pregnancy reduction involves the direct or indirect killing of living human beings.

Willke and other pro-life authorities argue that, once the respect and value of human life is cheapened, then nothing is wrong and everything becomes acceptable in the name of medicine.

Roe v. Wade Decision

Willke blames the 1973 *Roe v. Wade* Supreme Court decision as the root cause for this widespread acceptance of human experimentation at all stages of life.

"This thing is exploding all around us. The core, the absolute core problem is the *Roe v. Wade* decision. What it does is give an absolute property right to a mother who is pregnant.

"The baby has no absolute civil rights, no value at all. It is the property of the owner, and the owner can dispose of this piece of property in any way she wishes.

"What that has done is to take an entire class of humans and reduce them to a value of things."

Loss of Judeo-Christian Ethic

Dr. Willke also cites the loss of the Judeo-Christian ethic within society as the main reason for such a cheap view of mankind.

"It doesn't matter if it's human life to many of these doctors. They simply don't care. There is no respect for life. The basic reason I believe is the whole concept of loss of the Judeo-Christian identification, knowledge and belief. . . ."

An Immense Abyss

Bernard Nathanson, an obstetrician and gynecologist and former director of the Center for Reproductive and Sexual Health, strongly believes that a change in society's moral structure will be the only force to restrict such abhorrent practices.

In addition, he vehemently warns that, unless the public comes out of its lethargy toward such laboratory experimentation, it will only get what it deserves; and that is — being treated like laboratory rats.

"The general public does not understand the threat here and does not understand the clear and present danger which is implicit in all of this work.

"The abuses are so epidemic. The casual nature of this whole program with respect to its ethical question has been so persuasive. It is simply now becoming as institutionalized as abortion.

"Once you split out all of the ethical considerations from this, you end up with nothing but treating people as laboratory rats. This is only the beginning. We are on the threshold of this immense abyss."

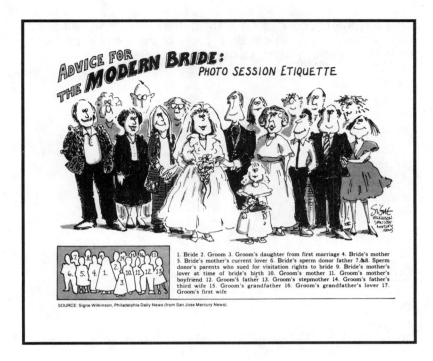

ADVICE FOR THE MODERN BRIDE: PHOTO SESSION ETIQUETTE

1. Bride 2. Groom 3. Groom's daughter from first marriage 4. Bride's mother 5. Bride's mother's current lover 6. Bride's sperm donor father 7.&8. Sperm donor's parents who sued for visitation rights to bride 9. Bride's mother's lover at time of bride's birth 10. Groom's mother 11. Groom's mother's boyfriend 12. Groom's father 13. Groom's stepmother 14. Groom's father's third wife 15. Groom's grandfather 16. Groom's grandfather's lover 17. Groom's first wife

SOURCE: Signe Wilkinson, Philadelphia Daily News (from San Jose Mercury News).

A Breeding Ground

Lacking any type of legal and moral restraints, Nathanson says, the future holds a frightening picture as the fields of genetic engineering and in vitro fertilization develop and the laboratory becomes a breeding ground for designing America's descendants.

"The long-term goal," he warns, "is to create certain biological classes which will serve the purposes of the technocrats. The potential is to insert animal genes into the uterus to breed an underclass which will do the menial tasks and chores of society."

Protesting Medical Practices

Other doctors have warned against the progressive nature of genetic manipulation and scientific inquiry. They have gotten the word out. Their warnings are clear. It is up to the American people to rise up and protest such medical practices.

If everyone chooses to do nothing, they warn, then we should not be surprised when certain aspects of the medical profession treat *us* as nothing worth saving.

MOVING TOWARD EUGENICS?

UNTOLD PROMISE:
THE NEW REPRODUCTIVE
TECHNOLOGIES

Robert J. Stillman

Robert J. Stillman presented the following testimony in his capacity as associate professor and director of the Division of Reproductive Endocrinology and Fertility, George Washington University Medical Center, Washington, D.C.

Points to Consider:

1. What are the two basic biologic laws applying to all species? What is the biologic purpose of the reproductive cycle?

2. Why does infertility appear to be increasing?

3. Describe the costs associated with infertility.

4. How are new procedures and reproductive technologies able to help infertile couples?

Excerpted from the testimony of Robert J. Stillman before the House Select Committee on Children, Youth, and Families, May 21, 1987.

41

The new reproductive technologies now hold untold promise and capabilities for therapy for the patients who had previously been unsuccessful at conceiving with more standard therapies.

I have been asked to summarize definitions, statistics, and the human and financial costs of infertility as a background to deliberations on the new "alternate" reproductive technologies. . . .

Background Information

The monthly cycle in women of reproductive age is comprised of a delicate, balanced, and orchestrated series of events leading to ovulation (passing of a mature egg from the ovary), the transport of millions of sperm through the female reproductive tract, fertilization in vivo, i.e., "in life" (as opposed to in vitro, i.e., "under glass"), and implantation of the early dividing embryo into the wall of the uterus.

If pregnancy is not achieved, the body signals the end of this reproductive cycle, and the commencement of another with menstruation, or the shedding of the uterine lining. The stage is set for a repetition of the orchestration with its critical biologic aim: reproduction. Indeed, there are two main, basic biologic laws applying to all species and espoused by Darwin: 1) that of preservation of the self, and 2) preservation of the species. The biologic purpose of the reproductive cycle, is of course, the latter.

The Increasing Frequency of Infertility

We are, in general, unaccustomed to viewing the menstrual period as a sign of failure of the reproductive system. Yet that is what it is to one in every five or six couples, or 15 to 20 percent of the married, reproductive-age population who are infertile, defined as a failure to conceive for greater than one year without contraception. That amounts to millions and millions of American couples (voters and consumers) involuntarily denied the fundamental biologic right of procreating and having a family.

The frequency of infertility appears to be increasing, and for various reasons:

1. Contraceptives, like the intrauterine device, can cause tubal blockage;

2. An increased frequency of sexually-transmitted diseases

42

also may block tubes;

3. An increase in the absolute number of people of reproductive age. More of them are seeking infertility care, as social stigmatization of infertility is diminishing;

4. Reproductive toxins are widely found, such as cigarette smoking, alcohol, drug use, and environmental toxins;

5. A delay in childbearing decreases fecundity (the monthly probability of conception). In the human, this monthly probability is quite low (25-30 percent per cycle—compared to most animals, 90 percent per cycle), and decreases significantly with age. Legitimate social and professional goals of women, along with effective contraception, delay childbearing but may have an unexpected and unwelcome cost to fertility.

A True Life Crisis

The health professionals entrusted with the care of infertile couples provide support—not just technologies, for infertility is a true life crisis. First, there is often surprise: "How ironic it was to practice birth control for years and to have been infertile all along." Then denial and isolation: "I can't go near my pregnant friends, baby showers, and my mother-in-law." Anger, guilt, and feelings of unworthiness often follow. Masculine and feminine self identities are sorely pressed with infertility, so intimately tied to sexuality and to sex itself. Depression, and then grieving often are final stages in the couples' infertility crisis —for some, preceding a resolution.

Infertile couples, unfortunately, grieve alone, for society does not recognize or support grieving for a potential life. Therefore, even the couples' grief, since felt alone and without support, is unrewarding.

The Costs of Infertility

That is in part the human cost, the cost of unfulfilled dreams. There are logistical and financial costs as well. For those couples who can afford it, dollars spent are just another burden to be borne at the "cost" of being infertile. For those couples who cannot afford it, they feel further robbed of their own fundamental right to procreate, with help now being denied them simply because they are poor.

There are innumerable ways to estimate financial costs of infertility—summing cost of each test or the cost of each therapy; cost it takes to achieve one pregnancy among a group of infertile couples; cost compared to adoption; insurable vs. non-insurable costs, etc. The "average" infertility workup may be completed in from four to six months, at an average cost of $2,500-$4,000. However, the range is *much* wider—for a $50 semen count might clearly reveal a diagnosis, or the diagnosis may remain obscure even after several thousands of dollars of evaluation. Similarly, the cost of therapy varies widely. Therapy can be successful with $20 worth of an ovulation stimulant for one month, or require several surgeries of several thousands of dollars each. In vitro fertilization (IVF) costs an average of $3,500-$4,500 per cycle and may require one, two, three, or more cycles to succeed.

An Infertility Diagnosis

A diagnosis can be established in approximately 85-90 percent of couples undergoing an infertility investigation. The remaining 10 to 15 percent of infertile couples thus have "infertility of unknown origin," i.e., where no cause or diagnosis can be assigned and where diagnostic sophistication still needs to improve. Of the 85-90 percent of couples in whom we can make a diagnosis, male factor, i.e., infertility based on the sperm number or motion, accounts for about 35 to 40 percent. Female factors account for about 40 percent of infertility. These female factors are divided among factors which may influence the ability to ovulate, tubal function, cervical, uterine, or immunologic factors, as well as a common disorder called endometriosis. Of

44

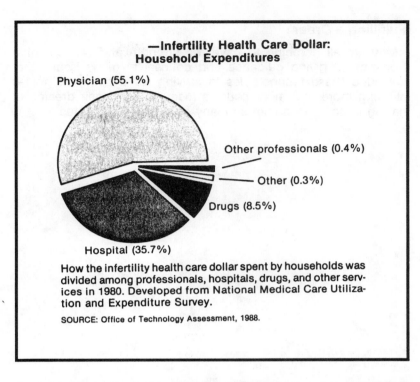

—Infertility Health Care Dollar: Household Expenditures

Physician (55.1%)

Other professionals (0.4%)

Other (0.3%)

Drugs (8.5%)

Hospital (35.7%)

How the infertility health care dollar spent by households was divided among professionals, hospitals, drugs, and other services in 1980. Developed from National Medical Care Utilization and Expenditure Survey.

SOURCE: Office of Technology Assessment, 1988.

the remaining couples in whom a diagnosis can be established 25 percent have a combination of factors ("multifactorial") causing their infertility.

The New Reproductive Technologies

Many new procedures and new drugs have expanded the number of couples whom we can treat successfully to over 50 percent of those who come for care, even before employing "alternate reproductive technology." Of the others, some may conceive spontaneously over time, others never. The new reproductive technologies now hold untold promise and capabilities for therapy for the patients who had previously been unsuccessful at conceiving with more standard therapies. Estimates of the percentage of patients who may benefit from IVF who were previously *not treatable* range from 80 percent of patients with tubal factor infertility, to over 25 percent of patients with infertility of unknown origin. Endometriosis, male factor, and immunologic infertility are also treated by the new technologies after other methods have failed.

Fulfilling a Dream

May we all combine to have the strength and wisdom of a Solomon in giving guidance and counsel in many issues that surround these technologies in striving for a common goal—allowing more and more couples today to fulfill their dreams of having a family—a dream so many of us take for granted.

SEX SELECTION AND FETAL TESTING

This activity may be used as an individualized study guide for students in libraries and resource centers or as a discussion catalyst in small group and classroom discussions.

DEFINING THE ISSUE

Modern bio-medical science has developed genetic tests to determine whether fetuses suffer from genetic diseases and other problems. The sex of the child can also be determined by this testing. Prenatal testing includes amniocentesis, blood tests, ultrasound imaging and others that help test for congenital diseases and physical deformities including spina bifida, Down's syndrome and other defects. An inexpensive and safe method of sex selection before conception has been tested in the laboratory. This procedure involves separating X-bearing (female) from Y-bearing (male) sperm in the laboratory. This procedure has been used at least once by an infertility clinic.

IDEAS IN CONFLICT

Outlaw Sex Selection Tests. Most people favor abortion under extreme conditions only. It is not moral to destroy a human life because the fetus has a medical or physical problem. Certainly no one can justify destroying an unborn baby because of gender. Gender selection violates the principle of male-female equality and should be outlawed.

Don't Ban Genetic Testing. Genetic testing of the fetus is a valuable tool that should be used wisely but not banned. These tests can help parents prepare psychologically for abnormal children, help detect and treat disease early, and in some extreme cases lead to a justified abortion. Genetic testing, however, should never be used to select the sex of a child.

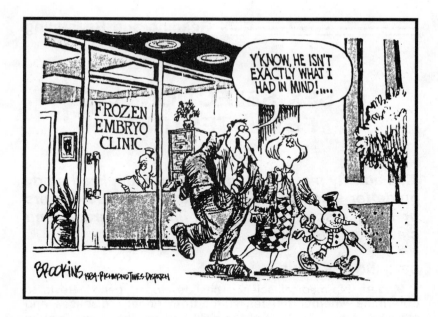

Sex Balance Is Not a Problem.   The ability to determine the sex of a child before conception is a great benefit to society. Those fearing that most couples will choose a first born male are misguided.   More couples (52 percent) choose first born girls.   Morally it is better to select the sex of a child before conception which could eliminate many abortions and the actual killing of babies in countries like India and China.

Guidelines (Part A)

1. Examine the IDEAS IN CONFLICT above.

2. Which argument do you agree with more and why?

3.   Do any of the arguments above represent an example of sex bias—sex bias is the expression of dislike for and/or feeling of superiority over a person because of gender or sexual preference.

Guidelines (Part B)

Evaluate the statements below by using the method indicated.

- **Mark the letter [S] in front of any sentence that is an example of sex bias. Mark the letter [N] in front of any sentence that is not an example of sex bias.**

1. Abortion is a private matter and a woman may choose gender selection as a reason to abort.

2. Sex selection tests are more humane than abortion and infanticide, which are used in China and India today.

3. All through history, boys have been preferred over girls in many cultures. Banning sex selections tests will not change that attitude wherever it exists in modern societies.

4. Sex selection tests that lead to abortion should be banned.

5. Abortion is an absolute right and we must live with the consequences.

6. A woman does not have the moral right to kill her baby because she prefers a child of a particular sex.

7. Many people believe that because something is legal it is right.

8. In extreme cases of abnormality, it is morally and legally right for a woman to choose abortion.

9. Sex selection tests before conception should be banned.

10. All genetic testing used on the fetus after conception should be banned.

11. Modern science has presented society with monstrous ethical and moral dilemmas that people are not yet able to confront with insight and understanding.

12. Modern testing procedures should never be used to select the sex of children. Gender is not a disease and genetic testing should only be used to prevent extreme illness.

13. Sex selection violates the principle of male-female equality.

14. Couples should have the right to have a sex-selected child.

15. Sex selection should be part of reproductive freedom in a democratic society.

CHAPTER 3

ALTERNATIVE REPRODUCTIVE TECHNOLOGIES

6 ALTERNATIVE REPRODUCTIVE TECHNOLOGIES

UNNATURAL SELECTION

Gena Corea

Gena Corea is the author of The Mother Machine: Reproductive Technologies from Artificial Insemination to Artificial Wombs *and* The Hidden Malpractice *(Harper and Row, 1985). She wrote this article in her capacity as the U.S. contact for the Feminist International Network of Resistance to Reproductive and Genetic Engineering (FINRRAGE).*

Points to Consider:

1. Define the term "technodoc."

2. Describe the disturbing aspects of reproductive technologies.

3. How successful is in vitro fertilization?

4. Why are women organizing a resistance movement against reproductive technologies?

Gena Corea, "Unnatural Selection: The Menace of High-Tech Motherhood," *The Progressive,* January 1986, pp. 22-24. Reprinted by permission from *The Progressive,* 409 East Main Street, Madison, WI 53703.

A growing number of women around the world see the threat the new reproductive technologies pose to women as a class.

The media accounts of new reproductive technologies all tell the same story of infertile women pleading with physicians who, prompted by compassion for the suffering of these would-be mothers, wave their magic test tubes and perform miracles. Women enter the clinics, become pregnant, give birth, and live happily ever after.

The "Technodocs"

In the already immensely powerful medical establishment, a new tier of experts is beginning to hold sway. These are the "technodocs," as Dr. Alan De Cherney, clinic director of Yale University's In Vitro Fertilization (IVF) program, calls them. Physicians and scientists continually expand the technology—always, they say, to relieve human suffering. They use donor sperm with IVF and, more rarely, donor eggs. They freeze human embryos. At least one—British IVF pioneer Robert Edwards—has announced plans to divide embryos.

Entrepreneurs in the United States view these developments as potential bonanzas. Some firms are offering to rent breeders, called surrogate mothers, to paying customers. One company plans to provide the embryo transfer "service" in a network of clinics around the country. This entails artificially inseminating women, flushing embryos out of them, and transferring those embryos to other women—a procedure fraught with risk for all the women involved. Other firms are starting sex predetermination clinics for clients who insist on raising boy babies.

Everybody is happy with these new options for parenthood, or so it would seem. But beneath the media gloss lies a profoundly disturbing reality.

An Attack on Women

As technodocs decide which women's genes are superior and which are inferior, who may reproduce and who is not "healthy" enough to, they distance women still further from our bodies, our selves. Future generations of women, growing up in a world of male-run reproductive industries, will have no sense of themselves as beings capable of procreating. They will know that women provide only the raw materials from which men manufacture people to desired specifications. In this sense, the

52

new reproductive technologies constitute an attack on women at a very deep level. At the level of consciousness. Our identity.

What's more, in buying and selling parts of women's bodies (eggs, wombs, hormones) in a new institution of reproductive prostitution, the technodocs and their business colleagues expose women to physical and psychological risks—risks that are hidden behind the smile of the happy mother.

If successful on a grand scale, they could intensify the class system: poor women, here and in the Third World, would serve primarily to carry the embryos of the upper class, and males would far outnumber females.

Control of Human Evolution

Yet another aspect of the disturbing reality behind the media gloss is this: such new reproductive technologies as embryo freezing, gene therapy, and the sexing of embryos provide a way to control evolution. Dr. Richard Seed, a pioneer in the development of the embryo flushing and transfer procedure, predicts that the technologies will start out as infertility treatment but will indeed eventually be used for the control of human evolution. He sees this trend as positive.

When reproductive technologies are introduced, they are presented as solutions to the problems of a small number of women. Then, quickly, physicians expand the indications and enlarge the number of patients. In obstetrics, for example, electronic fetal monitoring was introduced for use on women in high-risk pregnancies. Now, in many industrialized countries, it is used in most cases. The same pattern is evident with ultrasound, amniocentesis, Caesarean section, and genetic testing and counseling.

This technological imperative is likely to prevail with in vitro fertilization, egg donation, sex predetermination, and embryo evaluation. In vitro fertilization was originally proposed for use only on women who were infertile because of blocked or absent fallopian tubes. But physicians quickly extended IVF so that now even fertile women married to men with low sperm counts are counted among IVF candidates. Indications for the procedure continue to grow.

Producing Genetically Healthier People

Richard Seed says embryo evaluation may become part of routine prenatal care. Embryos would be flushed out of every pregnant woman and evaluated. Only "healthy" embryos would be transferred back into women; the others would be discarded. Some physicians have suggested that in the near future, people may use the sperm and eggs of other, genetically healthier people.

"Already we have had couples come and ask us if a male other than the husband could donate sperm because they were not happy with the husband's appearance or personality," says Professor Carl Wood, head of the IVF team at Monash University in Melbourne, Australia. "Similarly, women have been asking for donor eggs because they are not happy with some aspect of themselves." Among those aspects were appearance and intellectual capacity.

Genetic Manipulation

Once the embryo is outside the woman's body and in a laboratory dish, it is available for manipulation, including genetic engineering. The use of reproductive technologies for such a purpose was predicted long ago. In 1935, Dr. Hermann J. Muller, a Nobel laureate geneticist, foresaw embryo transfer, ovarian transplants, the farming of eggs from ovaries maintained in cultures in laboratories, and parthenogenesis (development of an egg without fertilization).

These developments "would greatly extend the reproductive potencies of females possessing characters particularly

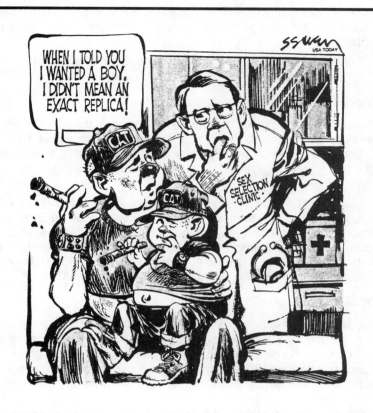

Illustration by David Seavey. Copyright 1986, *USA Today*. Reprinted with permission.

excellent," said Muller. "In such ways, and by otherwise controlling the development, the twinning, the size, etc., of the embryo, and the duration and other conditions of pregnancy and labor, considerable changes may be wrought in our methods and customs concerned with the production of children—changes permitting a much greater degree of control over our choice of these children, even before we reach the ideal condition of complete ectogenesis, or development of the egg entirely outside the mother's body."

The technodocs' suggested candidates for in vitro fertilization with donor eggs include:

- Women with genetic deficiencies.
- Those who have had several miscarriages.

- Older women who would like to have a baby but fear, because of their age, that they would produce a handicapped child.

- Women whose eggs may have been damaged by toxins in the workplace.

"Previctimization" Practices

Sex predetermination techniques may also translate sexual prejudice (a preference for male children) into a sexist reality. Dr. Janice Raymond, a University of Massachusetts bioethicist, calls this "previctimization"—the elimination of women before they are even born.

Previctimization has already become a lucrative practice in India, according to Mona Daswani, a social worker in Bombay. Doctors there have set up businesses to detect female fetuses through amniocentesis. When a female fetus is found, it is aborted, she says. Daswani estimates that 78,000 female fetuses were aborted this way between 1978 and 1983.

Population Control

Surrogate motherhood, a growth industry in itself, may turn poor women into paid breeders. John Stenhura, president of the Bionetics Foundation, Inc., which helps arrange for births to breeders, has predicted that once surrogate motherhood becomes commonplace, the price paid to breeders will come down. The industry can then go to poverty-stricken parts of the country where women would be more than willing to accept a fraction of the current $10,000 fee.

What's more, embryo flushing and transfer would open up the Third World as a source of surrogate mothers, Stenhura said. Using this technique, an embryo would be transferred into a breeder who would herself contribute none of the child's genes. Stenhura speculated that Central America, Korea, Thailand, and Malaysia would be appropriate places to find women who could gestate the babies of middle-class infertile couples from the Western nations.

This step would complete the already pernicious "population control" policies that are practiced, with Western money and supervision, in the Third World. Bangladesh, for example, has an incentive program to induce women to submit to sterilization. . . .

The technodocs are pursuing motherhood for Western, white, married women, no matter the cost to these women, and are pursuing sterility for women in the Third World, no matter the cost to those women.

Poor Success Rates

For all the puffery about these wonderful new technologies, the remarkable fact is that they do not work well at all. In vitro fertilization, in fact, is rarely successful. In the United States, a *Medical Tribune* survey of 108 IVF clinics found that half the responding fifty-four clinics have never sent a woman home with a baby.

All these clinics were operational and collecting fees ranging from $1,375 to $7,000 and averaging $4,085 per attempt. Of the twenty-six clinics which did produce births, twenty had five or fewer. Many of the clinics which have produced no test-tube babies at all or only one or two still claim astonishing success rates—some as high as 25 percent. . . .

A Resistance Movement

A growing number of women around the world see the threat the new reproductive technologies pose to women as a class. They are organizing a resistance movement.

At a meeting in the Netherlands in 1984, the Feminist International Network of Resistance to Reproductive and Genetic Engineering (FINRRAGE) was born. . . .

Last July, FINRRAGE held an emergency conference in Vallinge, Sweden, and women from eighteen countries participated. The delegates passed a resolution condemning "men and their institutions that inflict infertility on women by violence, forced sterilization, medical maltreatment, and industrial pollution, and repeat the damage through violent 'repair' technologies."

The Vallinge conference pointed toward a different approach to infertility. "Recognizing that infertility is often caused by political, social, and economic conditions, we support compassionate treatment of infertile women and intensive study into the prevention of infertility," the resolution stated.

"We support the recovery by women of knowledge, skill, and power that gives childbirth, fertility, and all women's health care back into the hands of women."

7 ALTERNATIVE REPRODUCTIVE TECHNOLOGIES

ASSISTING THE NATURAL ORDER

Gary D. Hodgen

Gary D. Hodgen presented the following testimony in his capacity as scientific director of The Jones Institute for Reproductive Medicine and as professor of obstetrics and gynecology at Eastern Virginia Medical School.

Points to Consider:

1. Have IVF programs been successful? Please explain your answer.

2. How does donor egg treatment work?

3. What is oocyte freezing?

4. Describe the three priorities for the Select Committee on Children, Youth, and Families.

Excerpted from the testimony of Gary D. Hodgen before the House Select Committee on Children, Youth, and Families, May 21, 1987

The public's trust in the "miracles" of biomedical research during the 20th century is the largest single reason for our successes in health care.

Introduction

Among the principal life objectives of most adults in America is the founding of a family. Having children in a number and at a time suited to the couple's plans and aspirations is highly desirable. Frequently, passing one's genes to the next generation is a strong motivation and significant part of the marriage relationship and family experience, as are pregnancy and parenting. However, the nurturing of children, youth, and adults within the structure of family can be compromised when severe developmental defects afflict fetuses, children, and youth. Thus, fertility, contraception, and congenital normalcy are high priorities for families.

These are powerful forces driving patients to seek medical services for human reproduction. Increasingly, the needs expressed by patients persuade scientists and physicians of the need for reproductive research in the laboratory and clinic to achieve success in infertility treatment, safe and reliable contraception, and assurance that children born into the family will be healthy. The accelerated emergence of the new reproductive technologies reflects these pressures in biomedical science and health care delivery.

In Vitro Fertilization (IVF) and Embryo Transfer (ET) and Gamete Intrafallopian Transfer (GIFT)

Since the 1978 birth of Louise Brown in Oldham, England and of Elizabeth Carr, America's first IVF baby, in Norfolk, Virginia, in 1981, IVF/ET has been matured from an experimental therapeutic procedure to an effective and widely applied infertility treatment. I have estimated that the current number of IVF programs worldwide is approximately 220, with about 75 active IVF programs in the U.S.A. Perhaps up to 50 additional IVF centers in the U.S.A. may be established within the next 24 months. Many IVF programs have been developed successfully in association with different types of institutions, including medical schools and their affiliated teaching hospitals, private clinics, and community hospitals.

Among well-developed IVF programs, pregnancy rates have risen steadily over the past five years into the range of 20 to 30 percent. In the Norfolk program, the IVF Team has achieved a

THE ULTIMATE GIFT

I can hardly explain the emotional change in my life thinking that I can give the ultimate gift to another woman so she too can experience all the wonders of being a mother.

When the first baby was born, I think we all felt it really didn't matter whose egg they used because each of us helped to make the baby by assisting the doctor's perfect catheter.

One of the best things about ovum transfer is that it is done naturally. The donor just goes through her regular cycle to produce an egg, is artificially inseminated then, four or five days later, has the lavage done to extract the fertilized egg. The egg is then placed in the recipient within hours. The egg is removed before that donor even knows she's conceived because her body will not go through any noticeable changes.

This is the next best thing to the natural way because the woman can actually carry her husband's child and she did not even have to undergo any surgery. This wonderful process opens a door for so many women who either cannot conceive or are afraid of passing on a birth defect or genetic disease.

Excerpted from the testimony of Cynthia Imhof before the Subcommittee on Investigations and Oversight, August 9, 1984

27 to 31 percent pregnancy rate consistently during 1985 to 1987, despite numerous very difficult cases referred to Norfolk by other IVF and infertility treatment centers. Using current capabilities, for each 1,000 treatment cycles about 230 babies will be delivered. Importantly, the cumulative pregnancy rate after three IVF treatment cycles exceeds 50 percent. An additional treatment method, GIFT, also has proven effective in some groups of patients, as developed in San Antonio, Texas, and Irvine, California. By the end of 1987 more than 5,000 children worldwide (nearly 1,000 of these in the U.S.A.) will have been conceived and born by these reproductive technologies. Noting that the earth's human population reached five billion persons in 1986, the new reproductive technologies now account for about 1/1,000,000th of the total human population living today.

Donor Egg Treatment

Donated eggs have been provided to recipient women either unable to use their own eggs or to women lacking ovarian function, but receiving replacement hormonal therapy to prepare their uterus for implantation and pregnancy. This technique was pioneered by research at The Jones Institute in Norfolk and is now used worldwide. Usually, donated eggs derive from generous consenting IVF patients having extra eggs that are provided anonymously for fertilization in vitro by sperm from the husband of the recipient woman; resulting embryos are then transferred to the recipient's uterus. Sometimes the donor is a close relative, such as a sister. More than 30 children have been born using donor egg therapy.

Cryopreservation of Embryos

Although in the Norfolk program we have not relied upon it, increasingly, embryo freezing is being evaluated as an adjunctive technique, both to conserve embryos and to reduce the risk of multiple pregnancy when several embryos may be available for transfer about two days after fertilization of the eggs. In Australia and Europe about 60 children have been born from the transfer of thawed embryos. Here in the U.S.A., the first such birth occurred in Los Angeles, California, in 1986. Although many IVF programs in the U.S.A. have stored frozen embryos, the technique is still experimental and requires additional research to improve success.

Surgical Fertilization of the Egg

Among couples seeking IVF therapy are infertile men who either produce a reduced number of sperm (severe oligospermia) or may have large numbers of sperm, but they are unable to fertilize their wive's eggs even in vitro. Results from animal experiments suggest that a micropipet may allow microscopic surgical placement of a single sperm into an egg, thereby achieving fertilization and embryonic development. Notice that establishing this treatment method would necessarily create embryos as a product of the research.

Oocyte Freezing

Having the capability to freeze eggs for storage and later use would obviate much of the need to freeze embryos, therein reducing the ethical and legal dilemmas inherent to cryopreservation of human embryos. However, some scientists are concerned that the fragile state of the egg's chromosomes

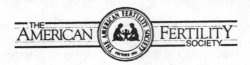

will make them intolerant of the rigors of freezing and thawing which could produce developmental anomalies. Thus, some investigators have advocated thorough chromosomal analysis of resulting embryos before attempting transfer of other such embryos for pregnancy. This raises the issue of embryo use for research rather than for pregnancy. . . .

Stewardship of the Public's Trust in Research

Ethical considerations of social responsibility in development of the new reproductive technologies have gained increasing attention in recent years. At the level of medical practice, there are questions about quality control for therapeutic services at some IVF clinics. Regarding research directions, there are questions about priorities, limits, review and oversight procedures, and especially about the respect and value accorded the human embryo. At the same time it is recognized that sound basic research should continue. These issues of public policy require even more attention when cost and fairness are considered in the restricted availability of medical care in the form of new reproductive technologies.

Three priorities for this Select Committee seem paramount: 1) a national policy on guidelines that provide some uniformity; 2) an enhanced dialogue between the lay public and the involved physicians and scientists so that ethical, religious, and legal concerns can be understood alongside determination of meritorious scientific studies aimed toward imminent medical breakthroughs, and 3) required availability of some insurance coverage to assist families of modest economic means to have well children and youth.

The public's trust in the "miracles" of biomedical research during the 20th century is the largest single reason for our successes in health care. As the stewards of this irreplaceable confidence, we must see that the public's trust in scientific research will be preserved for families of the 21st century.

8   ALTERNATIVE REPRODUCTIVE TECHNOLOGIES

PROHIBITING NEW REPRODUCTIVE TECHNOLOGIES: THE POINT

Donald McCarthy

Donald McCarthy presented the following testimony in his capacity as director of education at the Pope John XXIII Medical, Moral, and Education Research and Education Center in St. Louis, Missouri. The Center studies emerging medical moral issues from the perspective of the Judeo-Christian tradition and Catholic teaching.

Points to Consider:

1. Why does the author believe that some reproductive technologies jeopardize the values of the unified family?

2. Describe the author's six guidelines.

3. Explain why the author objects to freezing human embryos.

4. How does extramarital parenting violate the rights of the child?

Excerpted from the testimony of Donald McCarthy before the House Subcommittee on Investigations and Oversight of the House Committee on Science and Technology, August 8, 1984.

We are committed in our democratic heritage to protect the life and rights of the weakest and most helpless members of society, and I think embryos are members of our society.

Recognizing the Family

I think our nation and other nations have for centuries given clear recognition to the family, that is to married couples and their children, and this recognition flows from justice, that out of justice, the child to be conceived should be brought into existence in the context which best supports the child's individuality, responsibility, and sense of identity. And we recognize that stable families provide that context, even though unfortunately countless children are deprived of it, but this is the reason that we have a longstanding traditional effort to discourage illegitimacy.

Now, the same values of the unified family with married parents are jeopardized to some extent in the artificial forms of conception that we are discussing in this committee. I don't think the right of an embryo to belong to a family can be predicated on the sad state of family life that we frequently find in our United States today and the disintegrating instances of family life.

But I think rather the more appropriate approach is to ask the question, "Do we have a right to use scientific planning to deny the child's right to its own married parents?" Countless children are denied that right by the fortuities of human, modern social life, but put another way here, should our society cooperate through its scientific community in further undermining the family or in further denying the right of a child to married natural parents?

Can we prove from any data that in vitro fertilization from unmarried parents or that the triangle involved in surrogate parenting will further weaken family life? The data for this is not yet available. The point I am making is that such children have been deprived deliberately and with full awareness by all concerned of having both natural parents married to each other.

Ethical Concerns

It is true that adoptive homes are often more loving than the homes of natural parents, but that, again, does not annul the basic right of the child to natural parents. And if we are bringing children into the world through a technological procedure, it seems to me there is reason to respect this right of a child to his or her natural parents. In other words, I think there is good reason for saying that our society ought not collaborate in the injustice of deliberately depriving children of their natural parents.

Now, these reflections, of course, would even suggest the exclusion of male donors of sperm or female donors of ova. Artificial insemination of wives by donors' sperm is already in use in this country. The judgment as to whether legislation should restrict this practice or what might be done about the ethical or moral dimensions of this practice can be kept separate from our discussion today.

As I understand it, we are primarily concerned not about artificial insemination, but about human embryos, and we are concerned about the way in which human embryos are involved, in particular the lavage procedure of surrogate parenting, if we want to call it that, and, of course, the question of in vitro fertilization. And I am raising here the point of in vitro fertilization from unmarried donors of sperm.

I am going to suggest what I would call possible areas of legislative action or of guidelines. I am going to make a few suggestions in closing, at least suggestions as to how we might deal with what seems to be the more serious ethical issues relating to extracorporeal embryos.

Protecting the Life and Rights of Embryos

But in closing this discussion of the rights of extracorporeal embryos, I want to appeal to our American tradition. We are committed in our democratic heritage to protect the life and rights of the weakest and most helpless members of society, and I think embryos are members of our society.

We do live in an imperfect world marred by many forms of injustice, discrimination, and needless suffering. The point I would be contending is that the class of human embryos who are under discussion today, those generated in a laboratory or generated in a surrogate mother with possible lavage or flushing out and reimplantation, do have civil rights which need protection; that in a free and democratic society, we are called upon as responsible citizens to work for those rights rather than to acquiesce in technological violations of them.

Practical Guidelines

First of all, legislation or guidelines could, and I believe should, prohibit any form of experimentation on a human embryo which is likely to damage that embryo or to delay its natural development by delaying the time of its transfer and implantation. Only procedures intended to benefit the embryo should be allowed according to the ethical principle that we do not do unconsented experimentation on human subjects.

Second, any form of freezing of human embryos could, and I would suggest should, be excluded. The long-term risks of such freezing of human beings are still unknown, but even without risk, to subject human embryos to freezing, without their consent which is obviously unobtainable, violates the dignity of the embryo unless the freezing represented a proven kind of therapeutic procedure necessitated by the embryo's condition of health. I would make the analogy that we would not think of freezing perfectly healthy human babies after birth, so I see no genuine and ethically persuasive reason for freezing perfectly healthy human embryos.

Third, any deliberate taking of the life of an extracorporeal embryo should be prohibited as well as any neglect of reasonable efforts to implant such an embryo in its mother's body. The legalization of aborting fetuses and embryos in our present legal situation does not of itself entail the legalization of destroying extracorporeal human embryos or failing to implant them. . . .

More Guidelines

The fourth point I would make is that removal of an inviable fetus or embryo from its mother's body for transfer to another

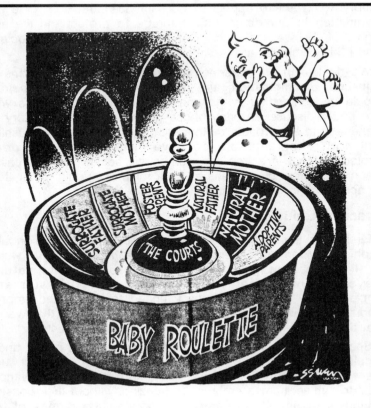

Illustration by David Seavey. Copyright 1987, *USA Today*. Reprinted with permission.

woman, the lavage procedure, could and should be prohibited by statutory definition as a form of experimental manipulation unless necessary to save the life of the fetus or the embryo. And if we cannot agree that it is a form of experimental manipulation, we might be able to agree that it is a form of exploitation of this tiny human being.

The fifth point I would make is that it would seem that statutes could and should insist that in vitro fertilization procedures unite only sperm and ova of married couples out of respect for the embryo's right to natural parents. The deliberate surrogate arrangement in which a woman brings to full term an infant she conceives from sperm of a married man for him and his wife also violates the rights of that child to natural parents as do all forms of artificial insemination with donor gametes and all forms of extramarital parenting.

We have made reference to all of these present situations. If the law tolerates these situations, that does not remove the inherent injustice to which I am pointing any more than legal toleration of other forms of injustice or discrimination removes the injustice or the discrimination. But I am simply not making recommendations about these latter practices, the practices of the artificial insemination, with donor gametes or even the surrogate parenting when the infant is brought to term.

The sixth point that I would refer to is that out of respect for the human embryo's rights, I believe the law could and should readily prohibit any parthenogenetic or uniparental procreation by cloning or any human-animal hybridization. No group of adults would seem to have the right to generate a human being by such procedures which include, of course, among other objectionable features the deprival of two natural parents for that human being if indeed it is a human being which results.

A Kind of Civil Rights Platform

Now, these six kinds of legislative protection or these six kinds of limits or guidelines to our manipulation of extracorporeal embryos could be supported and presented as a kind of civil rights platform for the minority rights of these tiniest human beings. I don't think these six recommendations that I have mentioned would eliminate all violations of the embryo's rights to its own natural parents. We know that every human being will not have its own natural parents, but I think at least these kinds of recommendations are desirable on the thesis that some protection is better than none at all.

As a matter of fact, there are many serious ethicists, myself included, who believe that the technique itself of in vitro fertilization violates the rights of human embryos from another perspective, on the ground that human beings have a right to be conceived in an act of personal self-giving and conjugal love rather than through a series of technical acts in a sterile laboratory.

9   ALTERNATIVE REPRODUCTIVE TECHNOLOGIES

PROHIBITING NEW REPRODUCTIVE TECHNOLOGIES: THE COUNTERPOINT

Lori B. Andrews

Lori B. Andrews presented the following testimony in her capacity as a research fellow for the American Bar Foundation in Chicago, Illinois.

Points to Consider:

1. How do the majority of people feel about surrogate motherhood?

2. Describe the government's role in alternative reproduction.

3. What does research tell us about the children and families created through alternative reproduction?

4. Why should legislators think carefully before adopting laws that restrict or prohibit the use of reproductive technologies?

Excerpted from the testimony of Lori B. Andrews before the House Select Committee on Children, Youth, and Families, May 21, 1987.

There has been much criticism of couples who use alternative reproduction. They are viewed as being selfish because they want a biological child. Yet that is a very human desire, one that is morally appropriate, and one that our constitutional principles protect.

Concerns About New Reproductive Technologies

The Baby M Case has prompted a vast societal discussion and has raised a number of legitimate concerns about the new reproductive technologies. Today I'd like to address those concerns and speak about the role of federal and state law and how it should develop based on what we know about alternative reproduction. In doing so I'll pay particular attention to the effects on the technologies on families and on children.

One lesson learned during the course of the Baby M case was that despite reservations that many people have about various aspects of reproductive technologies, the majority of people do not believe that surrogate motherhood should be banned, nor do I feel that such a ban would be constitutional.

A *Newsweek* poll during the Baby M trial found that the majority of people think that surrogacy for medical indications should be allowed and that the contract should be enforced. Similarly, a study by the Child Welfare League of America found that 64 percent of child welfare agencies favored regulation of surrogacy with only 24 percent favoring prohibition and 10 percent favoring no regulation.

There are also similar surveys about artificial insemination by donor and in vitro fertilization, which both garner the approval of the majority of the public. There is a strong societal belief in the importance of having the opportunity to be a parent and a recognition that for some couples the only way to become parents is to use reproductive technology.

Families Created Through Alternative Reproduction

The families created through alternative reproduction are particularly strong ones. For examples, there has been only a 1 percent divorce rate among the couples who have given birth to children using artificial insemination by donors as compared to the 49 percent divorce rate for the population as a whole.

The shared societal value regarding the importance of families, the fact that these families seem to be doing all right, along with the constitutional protection for the right to privacy should caution legislators that they should tread carefully before adopting laws that restrict or prohibit the use of reproductive technologies. Laws affecting alternative reproduction should only be adopted if they further a compelling governmental interest in the least restrictive manner possible.

The Role of the Government

I see the role of the government in this area as having two components. The first is to help assure that people have the opportunity to create families and in that respect I think there is a leadership role for the federal government in funding research in the prevention and treatment of infertility. The federal government could also enforce and even develop more laws to protect against environmental hazards and workplace hazards that present a threat to people's fertility.

The second component is to protect the physical and psychological well-being of the participants in alternative reproduction and, there, the primary concern should be the child.

The Children of Alternative Reproduction

Some opponents of the procedures, including at least one witness in the Baby M case, publicly stated that alternative reproduction should not be allowed because it is like adoption, and adoption creates damaged children. Such a statement not only stigmatizes existing adopted children but misrepresents the facts. Large scale studies have found that there is little difference in adjustment and achievement between adopted and

72

nonadopted children. A child born after surrogacy or donor insemination should fare at least as well as an adopted child, particularly since the child will be reared by a biological parent and his or her spouse, not a stranger, as in traditional adoption situations.

In the one area of alternative reproduction where there have been studies, with respect to artificial insemination by donor, the research shows that the children born through these techniques are thriving physically, emotionally, and intellectually.

The children born through alternative reproduction also deserve to have a clear indication of who their legal parents are. It has been suggested that the legal parent needs to be the gestational mother because gestation is the only key to legal parenthood. I think that's rather silly, because generations of men have been able to be recognized as parents without having to give birth, so I don't think legal parenthood should hinge on who gives birth. And traditionally, legal parenthood has been determined by statutory enactments. For example, in Arkansas there is now currently a law which says that if a couple contracts with an unmarried surrogate, that couple are the legal parents of the child and not the surrogate. . . .

Compelling Interests

Surveys about artificial insemination by donor and in vitro fertilization both garner the approval of the majority of the public. These statistics, along with the intense sympathy that many people felt for both biological parents seeking custody of Baby M, point to the strong societal belief in the importance of having the opportunity to be a parent. This shared societal value, along with the constitutional protection of the right to privacy, should caution legislators that they should tread carefully before adopting laws that restrict or prohibit the use of reproductive technologies. Such laws should only be adopted if they further a compelling state interest in the least restrictive manner possible.

The interests that are compelling at this point are the need to assure that participation in alternative reproduction is informed and voluntary, that the bodily integrity of the participants is protected, and that legal parenthood of the resulting child is clearly spelled out by law.

Statutes Governing Informed Consent Should Be Adopted

Society allows competent adults to take risks (for example, trying an experimental procedure, engaging in a risky sports

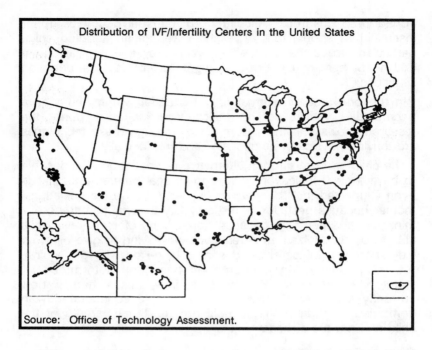

Distribution of IVF/Infertility Centers in the United States

Source: Office of Technology Assessment.

activity, or joining the armed services), even though an individual's decision might be motivated by a range of influences (for example, economic, social, or religious influences). In the medical realm, the individual is allowed to make risky choices so long as she has given voluntary, informed consent. Users of reproductive technologies, donors, and surrogates all need adequate factual information about the risks of alternative reproduction in order to make adequate assessments about whether they should participate in the procedures.

Informed consent of the patient is legally required by case law in all states before a medical procedure is undertaken. The legal doctrine requires that physicians disclose to patients, among other things, the nature of a proposed procedure, its risks and benefits, and the available alternatives. Patients have a right to refuse medical intervention. However, physicians do not have a good track record for obtaining informed consent generally, nor with respect to alternative reproduction. For example, infertility clinics generally do not reveal to potential patients the great variation that exists with respect to success rates. In a survey of 53 in vitro clinics, only 38 had successfully achieved the birth of a child. When artificial insemination by donor is used, the average length of time from artificial insemination to pregnancy ranges from 2.5 months at some clinics to 9.5 months at others. This points to the need for physicians to provide information, not about the overall success rate in the field, but of the particular qualifications and track record of that particular physician and clinic.

A law should be adopted requiring a health care provider to tell the potential user of alternative reproduction about the nature of the process, its risks and benefits, and any alternative techniques that could be used to create a child. . . .

A Human Desire

In the wake of the Baby M case, there has been much criticism of couples who use alternative reproduction, such as in vitro fertilization, donor insemination, or surrogacy. They are viewed as being selfish because they want a biological child. Yet that is a very human desire, one that is morally appropriate, and one that our constitutional principles protect.

10 ALTERNATIVE REPRODUCTIVE TECHNOLOGIES

STOP PUBLIC FUNDING OF THE BRAVE NEW WORLD

Henry Hyde

Henry Hyde presented the following testimony in his capacity as a Republican congressman from the State of Illinois.

Points to Consider:

1. What recommendations did the Ethics Advisory Board make?

2. Describe HEW's decision on federal funding of IVF in humans.

3. Define the term "selective reduction."

4. Why has embryo experimentation sparked such controversy?

Excerpted from the testimony of Henry Hyde before a House Subcommittee of the Committee on Government Operations, July 14, 1988.

We have begun to make Aldous Huxley's **Brave New World** *into a frighteningly imminent reality—a reality in which human beings are treated like products made to order, and quality-controlled by a technocratic elite that tries to make up in technical knowledge what it lacks in genuine humanity.*

I am grateful for the opportunity to comment on the current federal policy of not funding human in vitro fertilization (IVF) research. I will also explain why considerations involving the sanctity of human life argue in favor of maintaining this policy.

An Ethics Advisory Board

When the U.S. Department of Health, Education and Welfare issued federal regulations on fetal research in 1975, it specified that federal support of IVF in humans could not be authorized until an Ethics Advisory Board (EAB) had made recommendations to the Secretary regarding the "ethical acceptability" of such research. That provision was brought into play in 1978, when Louise Brown of England became the first publicized case of a live birth from IVF and American researchers applied for federal research grants to pursue similar efforts. But after almost a year of public hearings and deliberations, the HEW Ethics Advisory Board delivered to HEW what can only be described as ambivalent advice: Certain limited forms of IVF could be considered "acceptable from an ethical standpoint," but not in the sense that they would be "clearly ethically right." Rather, these procedures were "ethically defensible but still legitimately controverted" — or to put the matter in plain English, plausible arguments could be found for both sides in the ethical controversy. Among the unresolved issues cited by the EAB were the danger of abuse arising from experimental manipulation of human embryos, the "uncertain risks" to both mother and offspring, and the fact that the procedure remained "morally objectionable" to many Americans for a variety of other reasons.

I should note that the EAB's tentative acceptance of IVF was based on its view that the human embryo did *not* deserve "the full moral and legal rights attributed to persons." It admitted that those who promote respect for persons from the time of fertilization would necessarily come to a more negative conclusion on IVF, because the procedure involves so many risks of harm and death to human beings at the embryonic stage. But in the end, even the EAB "decided not to address the question of the level of the funding, if any, which such research might be given," because such a decision involved "scientific, political, economic, legal and ethical" questions beyond the Board's competence (*Federal Register,* June 18, 1979, pages 35033-35058).

HEW's Decision

This left the final policy decision to the Secretary of HEW. After receiving the EAB's report, as well as thousands of letters from concerned organizations and individuals, HEW decided not to pursue federal funding of IVF in humans. Among the most prominent opponents of such funding were the Catholic Church, some organizations of Jewish rabbis, and non-denominational groups promoting the right to life of the unborn. . . .

Faced with ambivalent advice from her own Ethics Advisory Board and strong opposition from many segments of the public, HEW Secretary Patricia Harris decided not to fund IVF procedures in humans, and this de facto moratorium remains in place to this day. I want to emphasize that this decision was made by an Administration and a Secretary of HEW that were not kindly disposed toward the concerns of the pro-life movement; if the same concerns are valid today as in 1979, an Administration publicly committed to the interests of the unborn would have even stronger reasons for continuing that moratorium.

Some Moral Concerns

My view is that these moral concerns are just as valid or more so today. As currently practiced, IVF poses several threats to the sanctity of human life.

My first concern is the role played by deliberate destruction of the unborn in many IVF programs, both before and after transfer to the mother's womb. Most IVF programs remove several unfertilized ova at a time from a woman's body, after using fertility drugs to promote ripening of several ova in one cycle; in some programs, all the ova are fertilized together in a Petri dish, but only the most promising new embryos are transferred to the womb while others are simply discarded. . . .The almost frivolous indifference with which this is done is one indication of a deeper problem in IVF: by turning the process of procreation into something more like the manufacture of a product, the technique seems to invite researchers to treat new life as a commodity subject to the most cavalier forms of "quality control."

"Selective Reduction"

In some IVF programs all fertilized embryos that seem to be alive and developing are transferred to the womb, but this also raises abortion questions. As was reported recently in the April 21 issue of the *New England Journal of Medicine*, this approach sometimes results in a multiple pregnancy that can pose serious risks to both mother and children. Some physicians resolve this problem through what is euphemistically called "selective reduction" of the pregnancy—that is, doctors use sonography to locate the unborn children they consider expendable, and inject potassium chloride into their hearts so they will die without endangering the one or two children they intend to preserve for live birth.

The currently available means for avoiding both these scenarios (discarding embryos before transfer to the womb or directly killing the unborn afterward) pose moral problems of their own. Either one freezes all embryos not needed for a particular reproductive cycle, which itself poses a very high risk to the life of the embryo, or one removes only one ovum from the woman in any given cycle, which greatly increases the costs

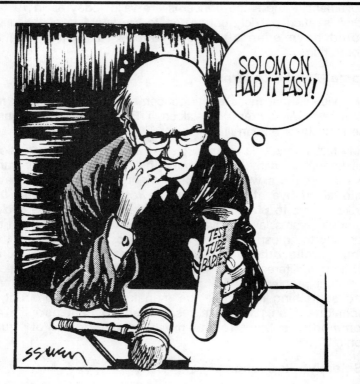

Illustration by David Seavey. Copyright 1989, *USA Today*. Reprinted with permission.

and risks to her because a new invasive procedure must be performed for each attempt at a pregnancy. . . .

Accidental Embryo Loss

Aside from deliberate discarding and destruction of the unborn, my second major concern has to do with the high rates of accidental embryo loss in IVF. Clinics promoting IVF often report "success rates" of up to 20 or 25 percent. Those reports have been called into question by medical experts who say the clinics mislead prospective patients about their chances for success; by their estimates the chances for achieving pregnancy from IVF in a given cycle may be less than 10 percent. But even if the higher figures were accurate, they would indicate only that a woman in an IVF program has a 20 to 25 percent chance of achieving a positive pregnancy test after the IVF procedure. To someone concerned about the loss of unborn lives, the most significant figure is the percentage of embryos that survive to live birth. According to congressional testimony of last May from the nation's most prominent IVF center in Norfolk, Virginia, that figure is 5 percent at best (or in Norfolk's case, 230 live births out of 4,500 embryos conceived). This is far higher than the rate of embryo loss in natural pregnancy. Judging solely by statistics like these, one could hardly call IVF an effective procedure for producing children—one is tempted to call it a fairly efficient procedure for preventing children from being born alive with a 95 percent success rate!

Embryo Experimentation

My third and final area of concern is that of experimentation on the newly conceived human embryo. It is no secret that much of the scientific interest in IVF has to do with the prospects it offers for new kinds of genetic experiments. Observing and manipulating "spare" embryos produced by IVF is seen as necessary for developing human genetic engineering techniques, and some researchers in other countries are said to have taken steps in this direction. This kind of harmful and non-therapeutic research violates the fundamental ethical canons governing experiments on unconsenting human subjects.

Ironically, some of the research made possible by IVF is itself designed to develop more efficient means for destroying prenatal human life. For example, the aforementioned 1987 congressional testimony from Norfolk's IVF center proposed that "spare" embryos could be used to develop new tests for a wide range of genetic imperfections in the human embryo, so that human beings who may develop mental or physical disabilities could be eliminated at the embryonic stage even before being transferred to their mothers' wombs. This project was described as a major advance, because elimination of the genetically imperfect could be made less difficult and emotionally traumatic for the parents than under the current practice of amniocentesis followed by second-trimester abortion. With such proposals, we have begun to make Aldous Huxley's *Brave New World* into a frighteningly imminent reality—a reality in which human beings are treated like products made to order, and quality-controlled by a technocratic elite that tries to make up in technical knowledge what it lacks in genuine humanity.

81

11 ALTERNATIVE REPRODUCTIVE TECHNOLOGIES

GOVERNMENT DOLLARS WOULD IMPROVE FERTILITY OPTIONS

Howard D. Jones

Howard D. Jones presented the following testimony in his capacity as director of The Jones Institute for Reproductive Medicine of the Eastern Virginia Medical School in Norfolk, Virginia.

Points to Consider:

1. How many couples have had their infertility problem solved by in vitro fertilization?

2. Explain how in vitro fertilization works.

3. What inefficiencies might be encountered during the in vitro fertilization process?

4. Describe the two scientific opportunities that need further study.

Excerpted from the testimony of Howard D. Jones before the House Subcommittee on Investigations and Oversight of the House Committee on Science and Technology, August 8, 1984.

It has not been possible to secure adequate funding to actively pursue research opportunities in the United States because of the policy of the National Institute of Health.

I feel that I speak for the 2 1/2 million couples in the United States who are involuntarily infertile with a condition which cannot be corrected by conventional means, but which can be corrected by in vitro fertilization.

Solving Infertility Problems

Since the first child was born, there are probably in excess of 700 couples in the world who have had their infertility problem solved by in vitro fertilization.

In vitro fertilization has been accepted as a standard method of therapy by the American Fertility Society, representing some 8,000 specialists in infertility. And guidelines, both operational and ethical, have been adopted by the Fertility Society and by the American College of Obstetricians and Gynecologists, representing almost 25,000 specialists. . . .

In Vitro Fertilization

As mentioned above, for many problems of infertility, in vitro fertilization offers a solution. In this process, one or more mature eggs are removed from the ovary by aspiration. The egg is given an opportunity to be fertilized by the sperm of the husband in the laboratory in a plastic dish. At one time this took place in glass (in vitro [Latin] means "in glass," hence, the name of the procedure). After insemination, fertilization, and after a period of up to 72 hours, the fertilized egg, now technically known as a conceptus, is transferred to the uterus of the donor with the hope that pregnancy will occur.

There are inefficiencies at each step of the process. By current techniques, it is now possible to obtain one or more fertilized eggs approximately 95 percent of the time.

The likelihood of successful fertilization and development of each of the fertilizable eggs is also quite high. This means that of all patients from whom an attempt to aspirate eggs is made, a transfer into the uterus of an apparently normally developing conceptus will occur over 85 percent of the time.

Inefficiencies of the Process

The greatest inefficiency is revealed after the transfer process.

When only one fertilized mature egg is transferred, the pregnancy rate is about 20 percent in our experience. While this rate approaches that of normal, it is certainly not equal to it and in order to improve the rate a great deal of effort has been devoted to recruiting more than one fertilizable egg per cycle by stimulating patients with suitable drugs and hormones which have been in use for many years to treat patients who do not ovulate spontaneously at all. This approach has been very successful.

With the transfer of two mature fertilized eggs, the pregnancy rate is about 28 percent. With the transfer of three, it is 38 percent, in our experience. The expectancy of pregnancy with the transfer of more than three eggs has not been definitely determined because the number of patients is quite small. Nevertheless, it can be seen that with the transfer of two or three fertilized mature eggs, the pregnancy rate not only approaches but now even exceeds the expectancy of pregnancy for normal human reproduction in any one cycle.

Facing a Dilemma

It is likely that further refinement will increase the number of available fertilized eggs. However, the transfer of more than one fertilized egg risks multiple pregnancies. While twins are medically satisfactory and socially acceptable and, indeed, often desired by infertile couples, multiple pregnancies above two do present obstetrical problems and certainly equally difficult social and family problems.

At the present state of knowledge, there is no known method of examination which allows us to determine prior to transfer which of the fertilized eggs will perish and which will produce a

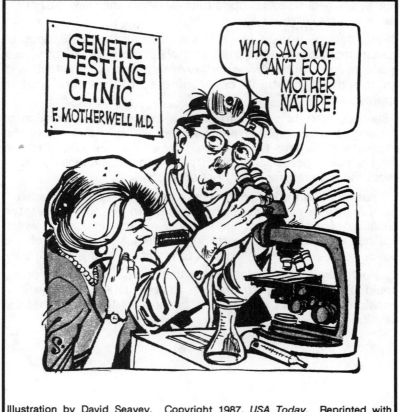

Illustration by David Seavey. Copyright 1987, *USA Today*. Reprinted with permission

viable pregnancy.

As we look at these eggs through the high power of the microscope, we are probably looking at, but unable to recognize, the factors responsible for the peculiar inefficiency of human reproduction. For the first time in human endeavor, there is an opportunity to study in detail this basic facet of reproductive biology.

The gynecologist and his patient face a dilemma. On one hand, to expose too few eggs to fertilization risks failure; to expose too many risks multiple pregnancies.

Two Scientific Opportunities

While there are numerous problems which need attention, I will cite again two scientific opportunities which this new technique has made available.

First, there is a need to study the details of the inefficiency of human reproduction. A solution to this problem would provide a quantum leap in improving fertility where that is important, and on the other hand, in controlling fertility where that is appropriate.

Second, there is a need to study a method of preservation of the egg, both unfertilized and fertilized, in order to improve the efficiency of in vitro fertilization by making it possible to repeat the transfer process for a given patient in subsequent cycles in event the first transfer were not successful.

It has not been possible to secure adequate funding to actively pursue these research opportunities in the United States because of the policy of the National Institute of Health, which will not accept grant requests in this area. The details of this policy are, I am sure, well known to members of this committee.

I would like to express the hope that in due course this policy could be reevaluated so that the United States would be in a position to offer its citizens the benefits of the latest medical developments.

ALTERNATIVE REPRODUCTIVE TECHNOLOGIES

SOLUTIONS FOR INFERTILITY ARE SOCIAL, NOT TECHNOLOGICAL

Wendy Chavkin

Wendy Chavkin, M.D., presented the following testimony in her capacity as director of the Bureau of Maternity Services and Family Planning of the New York City Department of Health.

Points to Consider:

1. How do infant and maternal mortality rates in the United States compare to those of other developed nations?

2. What percentage of American women do not obtain prenatal care in the first three months of pregnancy?

3. Describe the underlying causes of infertility.

4. What other suggestions does the author offer in regard to the new reproductive technologies?

Excerpted from the testimony of Wendy Chavkin before the House Subcommittee of the Committee on Government Operations, July 14, 1988.

Focus on new reproductive technologies represents a search for a technologic fix to issues with social roots.

I am starting from the presumption that our policy goals are twofold: that all Americans should be able to make choices about reproduction, and that we seek to promote social justice. The new reproductive technologies offer mechanisms for achieving one objective toward the goal of reproductive choice. Attainment of the goal, however, requires that we place these new reproductive technologies in context and the relevant context is that of a nation whose citizens too often lack access to *basic* reproductive health services.

Health Care Services

Rates for both infant and maternal mortality in the United States lag far behind those of other developed nations. Black infants continue to die at nearly twice the rate of white infants, and black women die in association with pregnancy at more than twice the rate of white women. Such racial disparities have persisted and, in fact, recently widened for these and other adverse reproductive parameters. It appears that the U.S. will not meet the Surgeon General's 1990 goals for infant and maternal mortality.

Because there is no national entitlement program for perinatal health care services, many American women receive late or no prenatal care. Approximately 25 percent of American women do not obtain prenatal care in the first three months of pregnancy. Because of geographic maldistribution of health services and financial barriers, other reproductive health care services such as gynecologic care, family planning, abortion and treatment for sexually transmitted diseases, are even less accessible. For example, 78 percent of all counties lack any abortion providers.

Underlying Causes of Infertility

The new reproductive technologies are geared toward increasing options for the infertile, estimated to be one in six American couples. Focus on these represents a search for a technologic fix to issues with social roots. I would suggest that we concentrate resources and attention on the underlying causes of infertility. Among these are:

- Sexually transmitted disease epidemics and inadequate contraceptive options. Pelvic infection resulting from sexually transmitted disease, and non-barrier contraceptive methods,

88

particularly the IUD, can lead to scarred, non-functioning fallopian tubes and infertility. Both of these require us to allocate resources for research, address financial barriers to health care to ensure that people receive treatment, and encourage public discussion of these matters to ensure that people receive correct information.

- Environmental and occupational toxic exposures that impinge on reproductive health. Lead and other heavy metals, pesticides and radiation are among those substances implicated in damaging male and female reproductive success. This requires a commitment to enforcing standards for a clean environment and clean workplaces that protect the reproductive health of men and women, and to allocating resources for further research.

- Demographic trends toward delayed childbearing reflect the fact that some women are deferring childbearing until their late 30s or beyond because of workplace pressures. Infertility, miscarriage and chromosomal anomaly rates all increase with advanced maternal age. Social policy must catch up with the reality that women of childbearing age are now permanently in the American labor force. Currently many women lose their jobs if they take off any time at all from work after delivering a baby. A parental leave policy that guarantees job security is a necessity so that women are not pushed to make unacceptable trade-offs between work

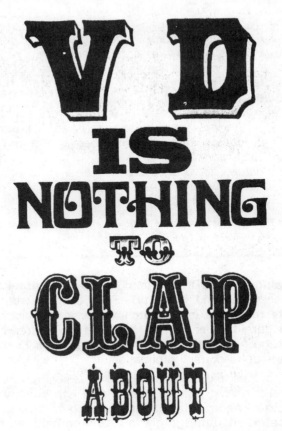

Photo credit: Library of Congress

Slogan promoting prevention of venereal disease

and children. Leave time to care for sick children and high quality childcare must become widely available in order to enable women and men to be parents and workers simultaneously. These policies would enable women to begin having children at earlier ages without financial sacrifice.

Rethinking Adoption and Foster Care

A second approach to addressing the problem of infertility is adoption. The questions raised by the new reproductive technologies offer us the opportunity to question our assumptions. Why are we taking for granted pursuit of a genetically related child in the face of so many children without parents? We could instead be rethinking our adoption and foster care systems so as to expand and expedite the opportunities for this type of family formation.

Watch for Social Inequities

Finally, I would like to urge that any new arrangements regarding reproduction not further exacerbate social inequities. As a physician whose experience is in obstetrics and public health, I am disturbed that some are viewing children as commodities and seeking to have the perfect child as they might search out the best refrigerator. A vision of children as consumer products extends to women as well, who are in danger of being viewed as disembodied uteri for rent or considered essentially as breeders.

Restrain Commercial Profiteering

To limit these more sordid possibilities, I urge that commercial profiteering be restrained. Our society already does not permit "free contract" when it comes to the sale of organs or babies, because we recognize the coercion implicit in the marketplace in a society of economic disparity. If we disallow fees for eggs, sperm, uterus use, babies and brokers, we reduce opportunities for economic exploitation while keeping the door open for medical innovation. Moreover, we refuse to allow venture capitalists to dictate our choices for research and resource allocation in this most human arena.

Until the social and health needs I have outlined are resolved, I would suggest that despite our stated respect for the rights to bear children and to privacy, material circumstances limit procreative choice for most Americans.

Gay Couples and Reproductive Technologies

This activity may be used as an individualized study guide for students in libraries and resource centers or as a discussion catalyst in small group and classroom discussions.

DEFINING THE ISSUE

Mark has fathered several children for lesbian couples through artificial insemination. Artificial insemination by donor has been widely used by lesbian couples in the recent past. Gay male couples may also use this procedure which for them is more legally complex since a surrogate mother must agree to be artificially inseminated to carry the baby to term and allow the male couple to adopt and/or raise the child. The gay male couple usually agrees on which one will provide the sperm unless a medical problem would prevent either from serving as a sperm donor. With the rapid development of new reproductive technologies both sex and gender can be removed from reproduction.

Guidelines

1. See how many factual statements you can locate in the seven items listed on the next page.

2. Which of the following statements do you agree with the most? The least?

3. Rate all the statements with an "A" for Agree and "D" for Disagree.

Statement one: People no longer must have sex to have a child.

Statement two: People no longer must be heterosexual to have a child.

Statement three: A child who grows up with a male gay couple is likely to feel confused about sexual identity.

Statement four: People must no longer be married to have a child.

Statement five: Gay couples are not fit to have a child.

Statement six: There have been no studies about confused sexual identity in children with gay couples for parents.

Statement seven: Loving care with a stable relationship is more important to a child than the parents' sexual identity.

CHAPTER 4

SURROGATE MOTHERS

ISSUES IN SURROGATE MOTHERHOOD: AN OVERVIEW

Reta Reimer

Reta Reimer wrote the following summary in her capacity as a legislative attorney for the American Law Division, Library of Congress.

Reta Reimer, "Analysis of Legal and Constitutional Issues Involved in Surrogate Motherhood," Library of Congress Congressional Research Service Report, March 4, 1988.

Recent advances in reproductive technology have made it possible for many previously infertile couples to become parents. However, the law has not kept pace with the evolving technology in this area, so many legal and constitutional questions raised by use of these new procedures remain unresolved.

What Is Surrogate Motherhood?

Surrogate motherhood is a procedure by which a woman is impregnated with the semen of a man who is not her husband and agrees to turn over the child born as a result of that action to the child's biological father and his wife, usually in exchange for financial considerations. Although many support this practice as the last hope for infertile couples to bear a child to whom they are biologically related, others argue that it is legally, constitutionally, and morally invalid and thus should be prohibited. This reading is concerned with the legal and constitutional components of this argument.

The "Baby M" Case

National attention became focused on this situation through the New Jersey "Baby M" case, in which a surrogate mother refused to surrender the daughter she bore pursuant to a surrogacy contract and thus breached the terms of the contract requiring that she do so. When the father sued to enforce the contract, a New Jersey superior court upheld it as a valid exercise of the father's constitutionally protected right to procreate, and ordered its specific performance — that is, the mother was forced to relinquish the child and her parental rights were terminated. However, the Supreme Court of New Jersey has now reversed this ruling, finding the contract both illegal under New Jersey law and void on various public policy grounds. In particular, it held the contract violated prohibitions on payment of money in connection with an adoption and laws which prohibit the involuntary termination of parental rights of a parent who was not found to be legally unfit, in this case the surrogate mother. It also held that the father's right to procreate did not include the right to sole custody of the child following birth, to the complete exclusion of the biological mother. Thus the adoption was rescinded, and visitation ordered for the biological mother. However, the court said that custody of the child, which is always decided on the basis of the child's best interests, should remain with the biological father and his wife, with whom the infant has been living for over a year. The court found that they will provide a more stable environment for the child, and are

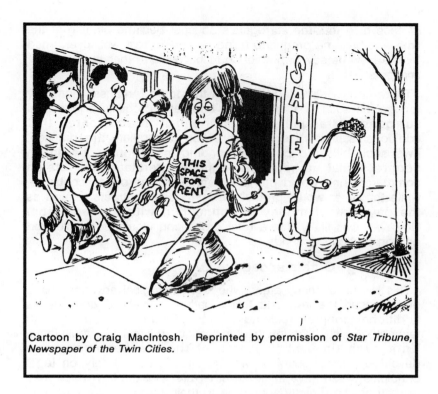

Cartoon by Craig MacIntosh. Reprinted by permission of *Star Tribune, Newspaper of the Twin Cities.*

likely to be more capable of helping the child eventually deal psychologically with the complicated facts of her birth.

Surrogacy and the Law

There is also a small body of other case law, much (although not all) of which finds surrogate motherhood contracts troubling. Two cases involve adoptions where the surrogate mother willingly complied with the terms of the surrogate contract; that is, she did not object to the termination of her parental rights or to relinquishing complete control to the father, so the courts had no basis for invalidating the agreement. Some courts have been reluctant to apply state adoption laws to this process in the absence of any indication they were intended to be so applied (which is unlikely, inasmuch as most were enacted years before alternative birth techniques were feasible, much less widely available). The Kentucky Supreme Court has upheld surrogacy agreements, but said that the birth mother has until five days after birth to change her mind; if she does, the parties are in the position of any other unwed parents vis-a-vis the child. In contrast, the New Jersey Superior Court which decided the *Baby*

M case held that the surrogate's consent became binding at the time she became pregnant, using reasoning that was overturned by the New Jersey Supreme Court but which other courts might find persuasive.

There is little state legislation on this topic (Arkansas generally recognizes such contracts, while Louisiana prohibits commercial surrogacy arrangements), although it is anticipated that additional states will soon take action to regulate this practice. Two such bills are currently pending in Congress, based on congressional authority to regulate interstate and foreign commerce; one would prohibit commercial surrogacy contracts, while the other would prohibit *all* surrogacy contracts as well as the payment of money in connection with any adoption. However, it is likely that a total prohibition would be challenged on constitutional grounds.

Technology Outdistanced the Law

This is one of many areas where technological advances have outdistanced the law, and this situation is likely to continue as additional couples take advantage of other alternative birth technologies such as in vitro fertilization and embryo transplants. Until such time as this area of the law becomes more developed, those involved in this situation must rely on legal principles which have arisen in other areas of the law which may or may not be directly applicable to their cases.

HUMAN SLAVERY

Gena Corea

Gena Corea is the co-chairperson of the National Coalition Against Surrogacy. She is the author of The Mother Machine *and the co-Latin and North American editor of* Reproductive and Genetic Engineering: International Feminist Viewpoints.

Points to Consider:

1. Why is surrogacy a public policy issue of enormous importance?

2. What is meant by the "industrialization of reproduction"?

3. The author says reproductive slavery is the real issue for women. What is meant by this?

4. In what ways has the surrogate industry shocked the public?

5. Who is Harvey Berman and what did he advocate?

Excerpted from the testimony of Gena Corea before the House Subcommittee on Transportation, Tourism, and Hazardous Materials, October 15, 1987.

The real questions are: Is reproductive slavery appropriate for women? Is this good public policy?

Surrogacy is a public policy issue of enormous historical and world-wide significance. That it is a public policy issue is evident from the following facts:

The Reproductive Supermarket

The rise of the surrogate industry does not take place in isolation. It's part of the industrialization of reproduction. It's part of the opening up of the Reproductive Supermarket. At the same time companies are being set up to sell women as breeders so that customers can get the products they order (babies), other companies are forming as well: companies that sell sex predetermination technology so that parents can predetermine the sex of their children (Gametrics, Inc.); companies that flush embryos out of some women for transfer into others (Fertility and Genetics Research, Inc.); and franchised in vitro fertilization clinics (In Vitro Care, Inc., IVF Australia Pty. Ltd.).

The new reproductive technologies (such as amniocentesis, in vitro fertilization, sex predetermination, embryo flushing) have already been used in conjunction with surrogacy and will be to an ever increasing degree unless there are public policy decisions stopping this. For example, let's look at some of the recent surrogate cases:

Some Surrogate Cases

1) Patty Foster. Surrogacy combined with sex predetermination. Foster's sperm donor ordered that his sperm be split, separating out male-engendering and female-engendering sperm, and that Foster be inseminated only with the male sperm. He wanted not just any child, but a son.

2) Mary Beth Whitehead. Surrogacy combined with amniocentesis. Although Whitehead was under 30 and not in need of any prenatal diagnosis, she was required to submit to amniocentesis, essentially for quality control over the product she was producing. She bitterly resented this and did resist it, unsuccessfully. (The contract called for her to abort if the test found the product not up to snuff, the only part of the contract Judge Harvey Sorkow did not uphold.)

3) Alejandra Munoz. Surrogacy combined with embryo flushing. Munoz, a 21-year-old Mexican woman with a second

grade education and no knowledge of the English language, was brought across the border illegally to produce a child for a man in National City near San Diego. She was told that she would be artificially inseminated and that, after three weeks, the embryo would be flushed out of her and transferred into the womb of the man's wife. She was familiar with the concept, knowing that that procedure was used on cows on farms near her home in Mexico. Several weeks into her pregnancy, she was told the procedure couldn't be done and she'd have to carry the child to term. According to Munoz and her cousin, she was kept in the couple's home and, for most of the pregnancy, not allowed to leave the house even for walks because the wife planned to present the baby as her own. When visiting her husband's family, she wore maternity clothes over a small pillow. Munoz, who had planned to be in the country for only a few weeks for what she thought would be a minor procedure, ended up undergoing major surgery—a caesarean section. She was offered $1,500—well below the exploitive $10,000 fee generally offered white women. She rejected the fee and has won nominal joint custody of her daughter. However, the child lives with the father and Munoz essentially gets visitation. There are constant fears that she will eventually be deported as an illegal alien.

4) Laurie Yates. Surrogacy combined with super-ovulation, a

procedure used and increasingly being developed in in vitro fertilization programs. She apparently didn't get pregnant fast enough, whether for the doctor or the customer is not clear. She was not an efficient enough manufacturing plant. (When I asked Laurie if she had had any say concerning whether or not she would be super-ovulated, she replied: "He [the doctor] *told* me, 'We're going to give you. . .' He didn't *ask* me.")

More Surrogate Cases

5) "Jane Doe." Surrogacy with super-ovulation. Between the ages of 14 and 25, Jane Doe had had nine pregnancies, five of which ended in miscarriage, Rochelle Sharpe of Gannett News Service has reported. According to Doe, when the physician who screened her for the surrogate company heard she had had nine pregnancies, he was not alarmed. Instead, he said, "Good, you're really fertile." Since she was breastfeeding an infant at the time she agreed to be inseminated, she was not ovulating. Instead of waiting for her to begin ovulating again naturally, the physician super-ovulated her with fertility drugs.

6) Shannon Boff. Surrogacy with in vitro fertilization. An egg was extracted from an infertile woman, fertilized in the lab with the sperm of the woman's husband and then transferred into the womb of Shannon Boff. She gestated the child, delivered it and then turned it over to the couple. (The reason the infertile wife had no uterus was that after becoming pregnant in an in vitro fertilization program in England, she had lost the baby during pregnancy and had to have a hysterectomy.)

7) Pat Anthony. Surrogacy with in vitro fertilization. Mrs. Anthony, a 48-year-old South African woman, was implanted with four eggs removed from her daughter and fertilized in vitro with the sperm of her son-in-law. She gave birth to triplets by cesarean section on October 1. Anthony's daughter, who already has one child, had reportedly had her uterus removed as a consequence of an obstetrical emergency. (The son-in-law, a refrigeration engineer said: "I couldn't be more delighted that my mother-in-law will give birth to my children." An IVF clinic director commented: "From an IVF point of view, I guess it's all over. It's really an obstetric problem now, and from that point of view I imagine a 48-year-old with triplets would be no picnic." (*The Australian*, June 4, 1987; *The Age,* Melbourne, July 4, 1987)

Going Against 'Laws of Nature'

Harvey Berman, the lawyer who took on the defense of Alejandro Munoz, decided at some point during his involvement

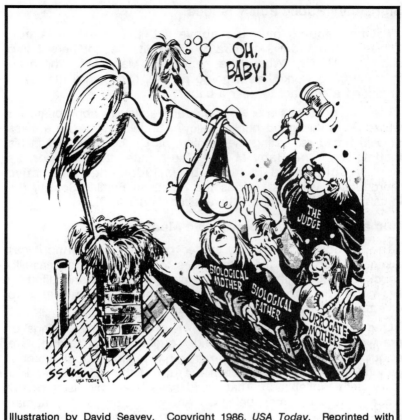

Illustration by David Seavey. Copyright 1986, *USA Today*. Reprinted with permission.

in the case that it would be a good idea for him to start his own surrogacy business. I interviewed him on this last April 24th. His plans call for using surrogacy with IVF, sex predetermination technology, embryo freezing, embryo flushing, and eventually, cloning. The physicians associated with his firm will use whatever technology they are developing, he said. Of his future clients, he said: "People that want to be certain what they're getting and are willing to go against the 'laws of nature' and get a product that they have chosen in advance—I don't see anything wrong with that per se."

So these technologies are being used, and will increasingly be used, in conjunction with each other. I think this raises the most significant public policy issues of our day.

Significant Public Policy Issues

To me, reading over the above list, the question is not: "What's wrong with Alejandra Munoz that she got herself into such a fix?" Or, "What's the matter with Mary Beth Whitehead that she once worked as a go-go dancer, had marital difficulties or signed a contract to bear a baby?"

The real questions are: Is reproductive slavery appropriate for women? Is this good public policy? Should we create a class of paid breeders, calling the women, as Dr. Lee Salk did in his testimony at the Baby M trial, "surrogate uteruses," or, as Harvey Sorkow did in his Baby M judgment, "alternative reproduction vehicles", or, as the American Fertility Society did in its recent ethics report, "therapeutic modalities"?. . .

Human Beings or Reproductive Meat?

The surrogate industry has existed only ten years. And it has taken no more than those ten years for this image to cease to shock the public: the mother of a newborn being handcuffed by five cops and thrown into a patrol car because she refuses to give up her baby to the man who paid for it.

One public policy question is: Are women human beings or are we reproductive meat? And I guess I'm not talking here about a special class of women. I'm talking about women, period. That could have been me up on that table instead of Mary Beth Whitehead. That could have been my sister or my niece. Are we human beings? Are we worthy of any human dignity or should it be stripped from us as crudely and cruelly as it was stripped from Mary Beth Whitehead? (Making mistakes as Whitehead sometimes has— is that an appropriate pre-condition for stripping someone of human dignity? Then mine could be stripped as well. Going over my life, I could match Whitehead mistake for mistake.)

Is it in the best interests of female children to be born into a world where there is a class of breeder women? How damaging might that be to the self-esteem of girl children? If it is damaging, does that matter?

The Industrialization of Reproduction

Another public policy question: As a society, do we want to industrialize reproduction? Is absolutely everything grist for the capitalist mill? Are there any limits to what can be bought and sold?

In thinking about all this, an image that keeps coming to mind

104

is that of the shell game played at carnivals. The barker quickly shuffles the shells around and you must choose under which one the pea lies. The public thinks the pea (that is, the heart of the matter in the issue of the new reproductive technologies) lies under the shell marked "personalities of people involved" or "new hope for the infertile" or "prevention of genetic disease and resulting suffering." But the barker/huckster is using sleight of hand to keep our eyes focused on the wrong shell. The pea is really under the shell cumbersomely marked: "reproductive slavery" or "industrialization of reproduction" or "reduction of women to raw material, to inter-changeable parts in the birth machinery" or "eugenics" or "control over human evolution."

SURROGATE MOTHERS

THE RIGHT OF PROCREATIVE CHOICE

Michael Balboni

Michael Balboni is an attorney at law in Garden City, New York. He was a former counsel to the New York Senate Judiciary Committee.

Points to Consider:

1. What three proposals are described for laws that would regulate surrogate parenting?

2. How is the right of procreative choice defined?

3. Why is the right of procreative choice not absolute?

4. What is said about the issue of paying surrogate mothers?

5. How would legal restraints and prohibition affect the practice of surrogate parenting?

Excerpted from the testimony of Michael Balboni before the House Subcommittee on Transportation, Tourism, and Hazardous Materials, October 15, 1987.

In the case of surrogate parenting, denying the use of a surrogate mother, may, for an infertile couple, deny an option of procreation.

A Fundamental Right

When the Judiciary Committee was contemplating proposing surrogate parenting legislation, we were faced with three options: prohibition, legitimization (or the laissez faire approach, as we called it), or a middle-of-the-road regulation approach. Our first task was to examine the decision of the Supreme Court in order to determine if there were any constraints on legislation in this area. We found that there were. The Supreme Court, in a series of decisions spanning over 40 years, indicated that surrogate parenting implicated a fundamental right which could not be prohibited.

The right we are talking about here is not the right to have a child, but rather, the right to be free from *unwarranted* governmental interference in *deciding* whether or not to bear or beget a child. This right, recognized as stemming from the right of privacy, has also been mentioned by the Supreme Court as being a right unto itself.

The Right of Procreative Choice

The first known articulation of a right of procreative choice was in a 1940 decision, *Skinner v. Oklahoma.* In *Skinner,* at issue was an Oklahoma statute which authorized the sterilization of habitual criminals. Though the court struck down the statute on vagueness grounds, the court also recognized that sterilization of human beings involved a denial of a fundamental human right: the right to bear offspring. The court stated, "this case touches upon a sensitive and important area of human rights. Oklahoma deprives certain individuals of a right which is basic to the perpetuation of a race—the right to have offspring.

It was not until 20 years later in *Griswold v. Connecticut,* that the Supreme Court announced a "right of privacy." The *Griswold* court interpreted the Fifth and Ninth amendments of the Constitution as establishing various zones of privacy, as these zones of privacy were necessary to give the Bill of Rights "life and substance." In *Griswold*, the court struck down a statute prohibiting the use of contraceptives by married couples. In doing so, the court found the decision to use contraception as "lying within the zone of privacy created by several fundamental constitutional guarantees."

The Supreme Court did not really touch upon the issue of procreation, however, until its decision in *Eisenstadt v. Vaird*. In this case, the court struck down a Massachusetts statute which forbade the sale of contraceptives to unmarried persons. The rational behind the court's decision was a recognition that "if the right to privacy means anything, it is the right of the individual, married or single, to be free of unwarranted governmental intrusion into matters so fundamentally affecting a person as the decision whether to bear or beget a child."

Infertility and Procreation

It is submitted that the right of procreative choice encompasses all forms of procreation, particularly when the persons involved are infertile and have a limited range of options. It has been argued that the right of privacy, however, does not extend from the couple to a third party. This is not my position. It is my contention that the third party, the surrogate mother, is not a part of the couple's privacy right, but rather, she provides the mechanism by which the couple can fulfill their procreative decision.

Furthermore, the constitutional right of privacy with respect to bearing or begetting a child, is not means specific; it does not limit one's procreative options to simply sexual intercourse between persons. In the case of surrogate parenting, denying the use of a surrogate mother, may, for an infertile couple, deny an option of procreation. . . .

Regulating Surrogacy

Entering into the area of regulation with the goal of preventing abuse of surrogate parenting and protection of the parties, and particularly of the child, is no easy course to chart. For instance, there is the issue of compensation. Critics of the practice, moral theologians, and feminist groups point to the exchange of compensation to the surrogate mother as being coercive, exploitative, and degrading of the birth process in general. There is also grave concern about the entrepreneur in this area who would profit as a third party to these arrangements. Though legislative methods are readily available for regulating these third parties, it is not so easy, however, to devise a mechanism to deal with payments to the surrogate mother.

Compensation Arrangements

One may look at the compensation to the surrogate and wonder, "since we don't allow compensation in adoptions, shouldn't we outlaw it in these arrangements also?" The problem with this line of reasoning is that, as a practical matter, the surrogate parenting experience has demonstrated that women are not willing to participate in a surrogate parenting arrangement without receiving some sort of compensation. Though not listed as the number one motivating factor, the compensation is an important part of the arrangement. The usual compensation that is paid is hardly enough to be said to establish a strong profit motive for the surrogate mothers. Ten thousand dollars for nine months' work is by no means excessive. Outlawing the exchange of compensation to the surrogate mother will, however, frustrate the procreative choice of the infertile couple since there is likely to be an absence of women willing to participate in a surrogacy agreement.

Such a result would work to undermine the spirit of decisions such as *Carey v. Population Services*. In fact, the court in *Carey* has implied that activity which is otherwise constitutionally protected cannot be denied protection merely because it is the subject of commerce. In *Carey*, a statute restricting the sale of contraceptives was deemed unconstitutional since prohibiting the sale was essentially equivalent to prohibiting the use. In other words, what the state could not overtly prohibit, it should not indirectly prevent.

Prohibition Is the Wrong Response

Aside from these constitutional restraints on prohibition of surrogate parenting, there are serious public policy concerns which militate against embracing the prohibition option. Illustrated by the current practice, laws prohibiting these arrangements are likely to result in driving the practice underground. Once driven underground, those motivated only

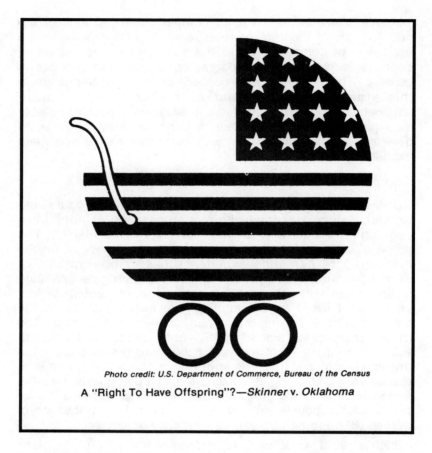

Photo credit: U.S. Department of Commerce, Bureau of the Census

A "Right To Have Offspring"?—*Skinner* v. *Oklahoma*

by profit will ultimately be the ones regulating these contracts. There will be no protection for the parents, the surrogate mother or, more importantly, for the children born to these arrangements.

During the three hearings conducted by the Judiciary Committee, over 50 different witnesses from around the country testified. Some of the more persuasive witnesses were those persons who had actually participated in a surrogate parenting arrangement. The sincerity and desperation heard in the voices of the infertile couples elicited a desire for a child with a genetic link and without the excessive wait for adoption. This desire is not one that will be easily extinguished by a legislative ban on surrogate parenting. Also, consider the 600 to 700 children already born to these agreements. What will be the effect upon them if we, as a society, condemn their method of birth as being against public policy?

Lastly, the New York Judiciary Committee acknowledged the fact that surrogate parenting represented the outer crest of a wave of new biomedical reproductive technology. We felt it unwise to allow our own fears and ignorance of new biological technology to force us to stick our heads in the sand and hope that these problems will go away. Unfortunately, the desire to have a child is something that will never go away.

Concerns Are Justified

The current practices surrounding surrogate parenting justify concerns over these contracts. The potential for abuse, exploitation, and commercialization are very real and should be addressed by the legislature. Prohibiting the practice, however, is far too broad a response.

Based upon the above considerations and my experiences, I am convinced that the best solution is to select regulation of surrogate parenting as the avenue best 'suited to protect all parties to these arrangements.

The Motherless Child: Where Did I Come From?

This activity may be used as an individualized study guide for students in libraries and resource centers or as a discussion catalyst in small group and classroom discussions.

DEFINING THE ISSUE

The egg of a woman—whose husband was sterile—was fertilized in vitro by a sperm from a commercial donor bank. The embryo was then implanted in the womb of a woman who agreed to serve as a surrogate mother for a fee of $10,000. After birth the surrogate mother gave legal custody of the baby to the infertile couple as specified in the contract.

Questions (Part A)

1. Who is the mother?
2. Who is the father?
3. Who should decide this issue and on what basis?
4. When the baby grows up what might its feelings be about its genetic origin?
5. Have we separated reproduction from sex?
6. Should the legal mother be determined by genetics or by who gives birth (the gestational or surrogate mother)?
7. Should we be worried about a technology that reduces pregnant women to the status of a commercial entity carrying babies to term for her employer?
8. If the parents in this case were forced to put the baby up for adoption, how would society define the real mother and father?

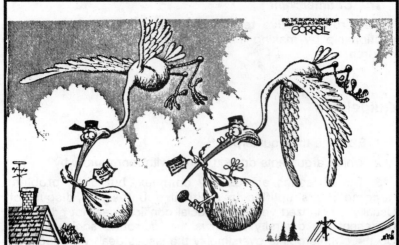

"Things are getting way too complicated, Bernie! . . . This morning, I accidentally delivered the wrong test tube to an irate surrogate mother who was overdrawn at the sperm bank, giving birth to a major lawsuit! . . ."

Illustration by Robert Gorrell. Reprinted with permission.

9. Has modern science taken us so far from nature that we will not be able to define the most basic of terms such as mother and father?

Counterpoints (Part B)

The Point

The terms *mother* and *father* in this situation should be determined in the court room.

The Counterpoint

The terms *mother* and *father* in this case should be determined by who gives birth to the baby.

The Point

The new reproductive technologies have separated reproduction from sexual intercourse.

The Counterpoint

New reproductive technologies strengthen the marriage relationship by making it possible for infertile couples to have children.

Guidelines

1. Examine the counterpoints.

2. Which arguments do you agree with more and why?

3. Social issues are usually complex, but often problems become oversimplified in political debates and discussion. Usually a polarized version of social conflict does not adequately represent the diversity of views that surround social conflicts. Do the counterpoints oversimplify the issues dealt with above?

CHAPTER 5

NEW CONCEPTIONS AND GOVERNMENT REGULATION

16 NEW CONCEPTIONS AND GOVERNMENT REGULATION

GOVERNMENT REGULATION OF NEW REPRODUCTIVE TECHNOLOGIES: AN OVERVIEW

Gary B. Ellis

Gary B. Ellis presented the following testimony in his capacity as project director of the Office of Technology Assessment (OTA) study Infertility: Medical and Social Choices, *which was published on May 17, 1988.*

Excerpted from the testimony of Gary B. Ellis before the House Subcommittee on Regulation and Business Opportunities of the House Committee on Small Business, June 1, 1988.

Congress generally does not regulate medical practice, with the exception of drawing broad criteria for care delivered at Veterans' Administration hospitals or reimbursed by federal insurance programs. Nor are medical techniques subject to consumer protection legislation, with the notable exception of Food and Drug Administration regulations for testing drugs and devices, and for regulating advertising of their indications and efficacy.

Regulating Infertility Treatments

Rather, quality assurance and consumer protection issues are left to state legislatures, professional societies, consumer groups, and word-of-mouth. However, some have suggested that the federal government take steps to ensure that infertile individuals are made aware of the efficacy of the treatments offered and of the success record of medical personnel with whom they are consulting.

This has been particularly stressed with regard to in vitro fertilization (IVF), for several reasons:

- Aspects of the technique are still to some extent in a research phase.

- Success rates vary considerably and even at their best are quite low.

- The procedure is carried out at times in free-standing clinics or other settings that are not subject to all the usual hospital peer-review practices.

- Relevant professional societies do not yet have accreditation programs directed specifically at IVF.

- As the procedure can entail months of drug treatment and repeated surgeries, it can represent a serious health risk and constitutes a major disruption of personal and professional activities.

- IVF is often excluded from insurance coverage, and so may be very costly to individuals.

- The patient population for these services is particularly vulnerable because it largely consists of individuals who have tried for many years to have a much desired pregnancy.

Quality Assurance and Consumer Protection

Congress could leave quality assurance and consumer protection efforts in the area of infertility services to the individual states and medical professional societies. Other medical services, such as novel techniques for cancer therapy, have similarly suffered from varying success rates and vulnerable patient populations. Without federal action, it can be expected that state quality control legislation, consumer education by private organizations, and medical society activity will attempt to protect patients from the risk, pain, disruption, and cost of undergoing the infertility procedure at clinics or hospitals without a demonstrable success rate. But such efforts will inevitably be spotty for at least the next several years.

By taking no action, Congress would avert bringing public scrutiny to a very private area of health care. It is possible that federal regulation of infertility services could change the character of those services. Sperm or egg donors, for example, may be unwilling to participate, and recipients of sperm, eggs, or embryos may be uneasy about medically assisted conception conducted in the spotlight of federal regulation.

Using a Consensus Conference

Short of regulating infertility treatment and research, Congress could exercise oversight to encourage the National Institute of Health (NIH), for example, to hold a consensus conference on innovative infertility treatments. Such a consensus conference — of which more than 60 have been held by NIH in the last decade — could be used to:

- influence the development of data collection on the use of IVF, gamete intrafallopian transfer, and other reproductive techniques;
- recommend the indications for use;
- establish conventions for reporting successful outcomes; and
- define standards for laboratory equipment and personnel training.

One important consideration regarding the appropriateness of an NIH consensus conference is whether the questions concerning the medical technology are primarily scientific and clinical, or primarily ethical or economic. The NIH conferences focus on the former.

Success Rates and Quality of Services

In the area of consumer protection, Congress could direct the Federal Trade Commission to exercise its authority under section 5(a)(6) of the Federal Trade Commission Act to examine whether advertisement of success rates at various IVF or gamete intrafallopian transfer clinics is misleading, and, if so, to issue appropriate regulations. Regulations could be issued, for example, to standardize the ways in which success rates are reported, so that individuals are better able to make an informed choice about whether and where to undergo a procedure.

Even such consumer regulation is not an effective means of directly regulating the quality of the services offered, however. Regulating a medical service itself—for example, by setting standards for personnel and facilities—would be an unusual step, as such regulation does not generally take place at the federal level, with the exception of setting quality control standards for Medicare reimbursement.

In addressing this issue, we are subjecting to public discussion sexual topics generally consigned to private conversation. But that is what is required if Congress is to treat fairly the estimated two million to three million American couples who want to have a baby, but who either need medical help to do so or will remain frustrated in their desire.

17 NEW CONCEPTIONS AND GOVERNMENT REGULATION

THE DOCTORS MUST BE WATCHED

Carol Peters

Carol Peters is the president of the de Miranda Institute for Infertility and Modern Parenting. The institute specializes in helping women prevent and treat infertility.

Points to Consider:

1. What kind of problems often confront women who use IVF clinics?

2. How can the de Miranda Institute help women avoid poor and unprofessional treatment at IVF clinics?

3. Why are couples unwilling to testify about their experiences with IVF clinics?

4. What areas of medical treatment need action on standards of evaluation and regulation of infertility care?

Excerpted from the testimony of Carol Peters before the House Subcommittee on Regulations and Business Opportunities of the House Committee on Small Business, June 1, 1988.

The medical community, which enjoys a special status in society, is not regulating itself.

The de Miranda Institute for Infertility and Modern Parenting (DMI) was founded in 1987 by Gina de Miranda and myself following a successful campaign to pass legislation requiring insurance companies to offer coverage of in vitro fertilization. . .

Our organization proposes to help the infertile by offering medical consumer education classes. We are currently working with Southwest Medical School to develop a course that will prepare the infertility patients for treatment by teaching them the rules of the road.

We are also collecting and disseminating up-to-date medical research. We hope to be a clearinghouse for this information.

We are publishing guidelines for infertility care.

Our long-term goal is to work to prevent future infertility by working with youth to prevent another generation of people from facing the same pain and expense that this generation's infertile couples have gone through.

A Confusing and Contradictory World

Infertile couples encounter a confusing and contradictory world when they enter medical treatment, and no one is selling road maps. We want to equip the infertile couple to make intelligent choices.

Here are some of the landmarks we tell couples about:

- Check physicians' credentials carefully. Look for board certification in areas such as reproductive endocrinology. If microsurgery is suggested, check for certification by the professional society of microsurgeons.
- Avoid OB/GYNS who continue to maintain more than 50 percent of their obstetrics practice.
- Get a second opinion, especially if surgery is recommended.
- Check take-home baby rates of any in vitro clinics if you are considering this procedure.
- Ask lots of questions and take notes.
- Avoid physicians who are unwilling to answer questions, appear insulted if you seek a second opinion, or refuse to make you a full partner in your treatment.

Infertility Stories

One woman who contacted DMI was almost blind after undergoing treatment with Clomid, a powerful fertility drug. Clomid literature clearly indicates that one of the side effects of Clomid can be visual disturbances and that treatment should be reevaluated if this occurs. Her doctor told her it was her glasses.

A woman undergoing IVF at a small clinic asked for a prescription so she could buy Pergonal required for the procedure on her prescription card. The nurse coordinator told her she couldn't do that because the clinic wouldn't make any money.

A DMI board member met a woman undergoing her fourth IVF attempt at a clinic that had yet to produce a pregnancy. When asked why she continued to patronize a clinic that had so little success, the woman said her doctor assured her he would get her pregnant and she believed in him.

More Examples of Poor Treatment

A DMI board member's chlamydial infection went undetected for eight years, even though she visited her OB/GYN every year from the time she was 16. Because of the infection, her fallopian tubes are blocked and she is unable to conceive except through in vitro fertilization. When she asked her physician why he had never performed a $40 test to check for the disease when he knew she was sexually active, he said it was too expensive to do routinely.

122

The day after surgery to remove an ectopic pregnancy, while I was still in the hospital recuperating, I was approached about in vitro fertilization by an OB/GYN who was opening a clinic locally. I was told I had a 25 percent chance of success, yet not one patient had been treated.

Another member of our board, who had patronized the same OB/GYN for years, decided to have a child. After six months of trying, her physician told her she might need infertility treatment. On her next visit she was charged $100. When she asked her doctor why, he said she was now an infertility patient and infertility patients take more time, thus the higher charge.

The founder of DMI, Gina de Miranda, was treated by an internist who called himself an infertility specialist. When she complained of pelvic pain, he told her that her husband was being "too rough." To relieve her pain, he administered steroids without her knowledge. To determine whether her fallopian tubes were blocked the same physician ordered a Rubens test. The test blows carbon dioxide through the uterus into the tubes to determine whether they are open. She was not tested for pelvic infection before the test was performed. Following the test she developed a massive infection and nearly died. It was only then attending physicians discovered she had chlamydia and that the test they had performed had spread the disease throughout her pelvic cavity. The group attending her then suggested a hysterectomy, which Gina refused. They then suggested in vitro fertilization as an alternative. Gina is at home this week recovering from surgery to remove scar tissue and repair damage done six years ago by inept practitioners of infertility. Only after extended treatment with antibiotics have she and her husband been cured of the chlamydial infection that surfaced so long ago. Her only infertility option: in vitro fertilization.

Fear and Emotional Pain

These are only a few examples. Since we began logging calls, we have been contacted by at least 75 people who are undergoing infertility treatment. Many are unwilling to testify because they fear retribution by their doctors or their insurance carriers.

Some patients wait six months for an appointment with an infertility specialist and they don't want to jeopardize their position. Couples in their mid-30s are fighting time. Insurance carriers required by Texas law to offer in vitro fertilization to subscribers have not only been doing handsprings to avoid

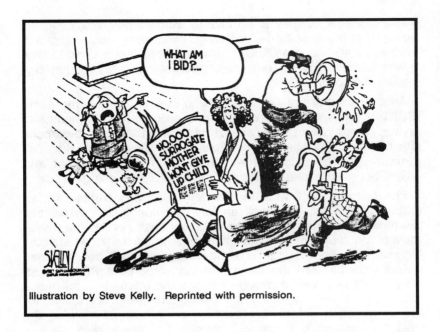

Illustration by Steve Kelly. Reprinted with permission.

complying with the legislation, they sometimes have penalized those who have made formal requests for coverage by denying claims on infertility diagnoses that had previously been covered.

I am offering testimony today on behalf of these couples. Because of fear—of doctors, of insurance companies—and their own emotional pain, they are unable to come to you personally. But Gina and I, who spend so much time talking to people about their infertility problems, know how too real their experiences are. They are truly victims.

A Regulatory Body Is Needed

How do we help? Education may arm some infertility patients to do battle in a caveat emptor industry, but it cannot keep pace with the exponential growth of the infertility business. In the last six years the number of women seeking assistance with fertility-related problems has climbed by 117 percent. There are 169 IVF clinics and their numbers keep increasing. Success rates, if computed at all, are more wistful interpretations than reality.

The basic in vitro process remains pretty much the same now as it was eight years ago. In Europe, residents pay about $2,000 per cycle for in vitro fertilization with respectable success rates. Established clinics in the United States, such as Northern

Nevada Fertility Clinic in Reno, report statistics annually and have controlled protocols. This suggests in vitro fertilization clinics can achieve the consistency of operation and control over cost that typify an expanding business.

Yet the OTA reports that less than half of existing IVF clinics have reported any success to date. These clinics, although operating as businesses, may be better described as ongoing, privately funded research projects with no overseeing regulatory body.

An Uncontrolled Growth Industry

This subcommittee must address whether the infertility industry will operate as a business subject to the same fair trade practices required of any other operation, or as a national research project, overseen by the government and governed by established standards of scientific experimentation. In either event, consumers must no longer be exposed to the naked self-interest of an uncontrolled growth industry.

If clinics are to be regarded as businesses, consistency of operation and minimum quality control, with a decreasing cost per unit as the business expands, are the least consumers can expect. Misrepresentation or poor service could then be reported to Better Business Bureaus, State attorneys general, the Federal Trade Commission, or pursued in court.

Classifying in vitro fertilization as research means normal parameters governing experimentation apply. Statistics should be reported to the National Institute of Health, for example, for dissemination to other clinics. In this way all clinics benefit from advances.

IVF clinics now fall somewhere in between. Although organized as businesses, many clinics are not producing a standard product. They are really conducting research, but without any of the normal controls.

Lack of Accountability

Consumers are caught in the middle. The medical community, which enjoys a special status in society, is not regulating itself. The least infertile couples can expect when deciding whether to undergo IVF treatment is dependable statistical evidence of success or failure.

Lack of accountability is one reason insurance coverage remains spotty and inconsistent. Unfortunately this lack of coverage has created a real catch-22. Without widened insurance coverage of infertility, clinics will never have the broad patient base necessary to widen clinical knowledge. One hand washes the other. And until some movement by bodies such as the Small Business Administration forces accountability, many hopeful couples will spend money they may not have to, and will undergo treatment they may not need.

MINIMIZE GOVERNMENT REGULATION

John Robertson

John Robertson is a professor of law at the University of Texas in Austin. He has written and specialized in the areas of families and procreative liberty.

Points to Consider:

1. What is common to all new reproductive technologies?

2. How does the tradition of privacy in matters of reproduction relate to a couple's choice of noncoital modes of reproduction?

3. Define the term "collaborative reproduction."

4. Why should state intervention in the area of the new reproductive technologies be very limited?

5.

Excerpted from the testimony of John Robertson before the House Select Committee on Children, Youth, and Families, May 21, 1987.

Many of the concerns are moral concerns or symbolic concerns, which may be very important to individuals, but do not form the basis for governmental intrusion into such important fundamental rights.

It is a pleasure to speak about the new reproductive technologies. And I think it's important to understand what is common to all of them.

The Tradition of Privacy

What is common is that conception is noncoital — it occurs without sexual intercourse. Noncoital reproduction, whether of the in vitro fertilization variety or whether of the collaborative variety involving donors and surrogates, is significant because it enables infertile married couples to procreate and rear children that are biologically related to at least one of the partners and often biologically related to both of the partners.

Now, in this country we have a long tradition of privacy, of autonomy of married couples in matters concerning procreation, family, and childrearing. It seems to me that this tradition of privacy in reproductive matters should extend to a married couple's choice of noncoital modes of reproduction as well. And what this means is that if state intervention occurs, it should occur only for the most compelling reasons, never on grounds of moral condemnation alone.

I'd like to explore this notion of procreative liberty a bit further because it's a centerpiece of any effort to explore policy in this area. And I don't think anyone would argue with the fact that a married couple has a right to reproduce by coital means. It's so well established that it's never even been challenged by the state in any way. I think we need to explore the implications of the married couple's right to reproduce coitally when they are not able to and need to use noncoital techniques.

The Right to Procreate

Surely infertile couples should have the same right to bear, beget, and rear children that fertile couples do, if the means for doing so or enabling them to procreate exist. A couple's interest in reproducing and parenting is the same whether they are infertile or not and as best as I can tell and estimate as a teacher-professor of constitutional law, I think our courts would agree with that when they are finally confronted with this question.

128

That means that restrictions by the state on noncoital ways of conceiving children have to meet the same high standard that restrictions on coital conception would have to meet, i.e., showing that the restriction is essential to prevent some tangible harm to others. Since moral condemnation alone would certainly not justify restricting coital conception, it should not justify restricting noncoital conception either. And this has important implications for an infertile married couple's use both of in vitro fertilization and assistance of donors and surrogates. Let me say something about each.

In Vitro Fertilization

With regard to in vitro fertilization where the married couple is providing both the egg and sperm, but conception is occurring outside the body, it would seem that they clearly would have a right to use such a technique, as against state prohibitions, if it is necessary to do so. This technique is now well established as safe and effective. But it's important to recognize that their right to use that technique would extend to such things as creating more embryos outside of the body than could be safely transferred; for example, if they get six or seven eggs, fertilizing all six or seven and then transferring back only three or four, which is necessary for maternal safety, and thus freezing the extras for use on a later cycle. And I think their right would probably also extend to discarding or not transferring those embryos that would present a threat to safety and it probably would also extend to donating excess embryos to other infertile couples if there were such couples in need, and it might even extend to use of embryos that will be discarded in some research for valid medical reasons after review by an institutional review board and other review bodies, if that is appropriate.

Collaborative Reproduction

Let me also say something about how this right of procreative liberty would apply to use of donors and surrogates, what I call collaborative reproduction. Obviously, no one reproduces alone; there's always a collaborator but here I'm talking about a third party collaborator outside of the married couple. And it would seem to me that if the infertile couple has a right to beget and rear children by the only means available that this would extend to making agreements with willing donors of sperm and egg and also willing donors of gestational services or surrogates, if that is necessary. And I think it's essential to recognize then that the agreements made with donors and surrogates concerning rearing rights and duties in the offspring of that arrangement should presumptively control. If the state prohibited such arrangements, refused to enforce the contract, or prohibited the payment of money to collaborators, the state would be interfering by making it extremely difficult or impossible for infertile couples to use these techniques, and thus would infringe upon their right to procreative choice. . . .

Interference with Procreative Choice

I've talked about procreative liberty as a fundamental constitutional right of married couples, whether procreation occurs coitally or noncoitally. Of course, calling it a right doesn't mean that it's absolute, doesn't mean that it cannot be limited in appropriate circumstances.

However, the key point here is that not every public concern will count as a constitutionally sufficient reason for interfering with procreative choice. The state would have to show some serious tangible harm to others other than dislike or moral condemnation of noncoital and collaborative techniques to justify interference. As a result of this constitutional position, it seems to me that both the power of Congress and the power of the states to limit noncoital reproduction is very limited.

Moral Condemnation

Let me give a couple of examples. The moral condemnation of all forms of noncoital reproduction contained in the recent Vatican statement would not justify state interference, no matter how strongly persons hold this view. Nor would a view that the embryo is a person from the moment of conception justify restrictions on embryo freezing, research or discard, again,

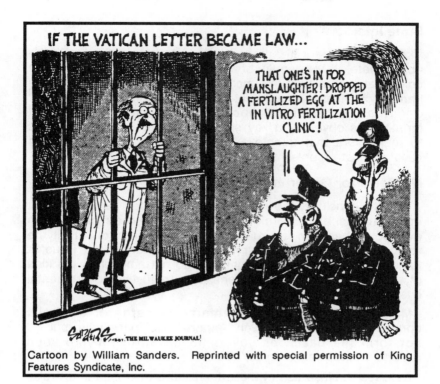

Cartoon by William Sanders. Reprinted with special permission of King Features Syndicate, Inc.

because that's a moral position that would directly interfere with procreative choice. Nor is the concern that is often voiced and has been voiced by the prior panel about commercialization. Commercialization may not be a good thing but the kinds of concerns that have been expressed amount to a kind of moral condemnation of commercialization and that fact alone without some further evidence of tangible harm to others would not be sufficient grounds for restriction. The statement was made in a prior panel that we don't permit the selling of babies and the analogy was drawn that we don't permit the selling of organs. Well, I point out, yes, we don't permit the selling of organs but we do permit the selling of organ transplants. For $50,000 you can get a kidney transplant; $100,000 a heart transplant and that sale includes the transfer of the organ and I think, that's an appropriate analogy here. The question of selling reproductive services that lead to transfer of a baby seem to me to have a parallel in the sale of organ transplants even though we don't sell the organs themselves. . . .

State Intervention

I think there are a few areas where state intervention would be appropriate. One would be to make sure that reproductive collaborators are fully informed, counseled and understand the transactions that they enter into because if the original contract does have legal significance as I suggest, then contract formation is obviously a key stage. The state could take steps to make sure that people are well informed, counseled, and have adequate representation at that stage. . . .

No Basis for Governmental Intrusion

Well, to conclude, the new reproduction does have important implications but I think to some extent they have been overblown because it's really a very small portion of all the reproduction that will occur. When we address the issue, it turns out that many of the concerns do not amount to the kind of tangible harm to others necessary to justify governmental intervention.

Many of the concerns are moral concerns or symbolic concerns, which may be very important to individuals, but do not form the basis for governmental intrusion into such important fundamental rights.

As a result, since use of these techniques involves the exercise of a basic procreative liberty, the role of government in regulating its use is necessarily minimal. As with decisions about coital reproduction, we must rely on informed decisions by the couples involved and the professionals advising them rather than the power of the state to assure that noncoital reproduction is used wisely for the good of couples, children, and society.

19   NEW CONCEPTIONS AND GOVERNMENT REGULATION

A STRONG FEDERAL ROLE IS NEEDED

Arthur Caplan

Arthur Caplan is the director of the Center for Biomedical Ethics at the University of Minnesota. He is a prominent international spokesman in the area of medical ethics and genetic engineering.

Points to Consider:

1. Why is the field of infertility treatment in need of federal regulation?

2. What is eugenics and how might it relate to in vitro fertilization?

3. How high are success rates for IVF clinics?

4. Why are the current procedures for informed consent totally inadequate?

5. What is the cost of the new reproductive technologies?

Excerpted from the testimony of Arthur Caplan before the House Subcommittee on Regulation and Business Opportunities of the House Committee on Small Business, June 1, 1988.

Infertility treatment is a field that is desperately in need of oversight, examination, and critical attention by the government.

Government Intervention Is Needed

There are many who have suggested that the best thing that could happen to the field of infertility treatment is that it be spared the ministrations of government.

I do not agree with that point of view. I think this is a field that is desperately in need of oversight, examination, and critical attention by the government.

We already have seen how desperate some of the consumers of these services can be. We have heard a lot about success rates. Let's not forget that the babies—which hopefully result from the use of these evolving technologies—must be heard and their interests articulated. Who is more qualified to do this than the federal government?

I want to say something about the aims of in vitro fertilization (IVF), something about the question of informed consent, and about some clinical practices that are questionable. I will conclude with a remark about research.

IVF Issues

One of the things we have to keep in mind is that our society has not sorted through what is acceptable regarding in vitro fertilization. We have been talking thus far about infertile couples.

The issue still out there is who ought to be able to use the technique, only people demonstrably infertile? Would we be unhappy if society turned to IVF as a way to create children as a means of convenience?

How about if the technique were used for eugenic purposes? Lest anyone think this is out of the realm of possibility, remember, there is a sperm bank in operation in California which has nothing other than eugenic goals as its reason for existence.

There is nothing about this that leads IVF to be associated with eugenics but it could be put to that purpose. If egg banking and the storage of eggs becomes possible we could find ourselves in a situation where this rationale will need to be looked at.

We should also keep in mind that the techniques can be used not only to create babies but, also, to create embryos for research. This is going on in some parts of the world.

We will have to take on the question of whether we want it to happen here. Two years ago I heard of a man in West Virginia who was in his eighties and had a large fortune. He lacked children. He decided he wanted to pass on his name and fortune to a biological descendent.

He wanted to know from me whether he could make an arrangement with an IVF clinic to create a biological heir. Is that a reason to come to a clinic? I am not saying there are a lot of situations like that, but that story should make us ask who should be allowed to seek IVF.

IVF and Informed Consent

Second, consider the experimental status of IVF. . . .We have independent confirmation that the success rates are not as high as some people are being led to believe. What I want to say about the problems of success rates basically falls into two areas of special concern we are beginning to get at today.

One is, in my view, that informed consent for the people who seek these services is totally inadequate. Fertility consumers are especially fragile consumers. They are desperately seeking any means to have a baby.

They will go anywhere, spend any amount, to have a baby. They can be preyed upon. Centers often give average data. To me that is simply unacceptable in the area of informed consent.

When one goes to a clinic one does not care about pooled or averaged data. One wants to know what is the success rate in this clinic at this time.

That must be provided, or informed consent is a charade.

Second, there is no mandatory reporting of data. . . .There is no requirement that data be provided in a systemized fashion by the centers.

Last, it is important to point out that many of these centers are paying no attention to a critical part of informed consent which is psychological counseling. That is not acceptable where informed consent is concerned.

A Legitimate Question

Another key problem that exists in in vitro fertilization is when do we pay? We have heard that some states have moved to mandate funding for in vitro fertilization. Some have questioned if the success rate is 6 or 9 percent whether public money should go toward this purpose at this time.

I think that is a legitimate question. Since the insurance companies don't want to pay and the National Institute of Health doesn't want to pay for what is being used clinically, the couples who are infertile find themselves in a terrible bind. The answer, whether from motives of fraud, malice, or good will, is to lie.

That is what is going on. We have a system wherein people attempt in vitro fertilization but no babies are created. The federal government has not taken a long hard look to determine when a procedure has evolved to a level of success that merits funding as a public program.

In vitro fertilization, transplants, artificial hearts, none of them have been assessed for efficacy.

Questionable Clinic Practices

The other two areas I wanted to mention are simply those regarding some dubious clinical practices. IVF success rates are so discouraging that there are some centers trying to do better in terms of creating babies by using multiple implants.

It shows at the 41 centers there were an average of three embryos used. There are many centers that use more than that. When they do, they sometimes create multiple pregnancies, three, four, five, or six babies.

Then they use fetal reduction, which is killing some fetuses to

136

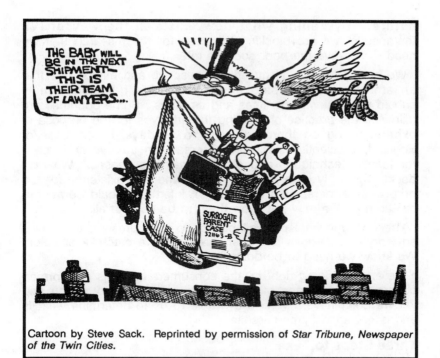

Cartoon by Steve Sack. Reprinted by permission of *Star Tribune, Newspaper of the Twin Cities.*

preserve the health of the mother and to help the other fetuses survive. That is a serious procedure. But because of the lack of pressure to standardize, routinize, and assure quality in the centers out there, we have this kind of dubious activity going on.

IVF Research

The last issue, an enormous one, more than I can describe in any detail, is the question of research in this area. I think it is scandalous that an ethics advisory board has not been appointed and no mechanism at the federal level has been created for approving research.

These techniques have to be made better. Sometimes you will hear it said that these rates are not bad because if you make babies the old-fashioned way the chances of success are still only 20 percent per month of people trying to have a child through sexual intercourse.

That may be true, but if you are using technologies that involve a risk and a cost of $5,000-$10,000 per effort, I think we should expect more from science than we do from mother nature. By calling what now exists in the way of IVF therapeutic, we are blocking the case for the research that we need to improve the poor success rate.

We have as a central question, I suspect, and maybe one that an ethics advisory board could settle, the question of how should we deal with gametes and embryos. Some countries are following the practice of creating the embryos for the purpose of experimenting on them. For up to 14 days, in the case of England, a scientist is allowed to create an embryo and use it for testing techniques and other research purposes. We may decide that only embryos that have come into existence for the purposes of therapeutic treatment of infertility should come into research or, we may not allow them to be used at all.

The only mechanism available to do it at present, the ethics advisory board, does not exist. We are in a catch-22 situation. We know we need to be doing better.

We are not doing right by the consumers in terms of informed consent and in terms of giving them accurate information and yet we don't have a vehicle available to us to determine what is and is not ethically permissible. . . .

Three Steps to Take

I think I would recommend three steps to be taken: First, we need to continue to pressure Health and Human Services to appoint that ethics advisory board. It should be appointed. It can be appointed expeditiously.

It can begin to wrestle with some of these questions we have been talking about before. It is not that the questions don't arise, it is not that the issues aren't there. The ethics advisory board is a forum where they can be appropriately debated or discussed whatever the ultimate resolution is going to be.

Second, I think we should be insisting, as I said earlier, that if there is going to be federal reimbursement for techniques like IVF, that certain standards be created concerning professional qualifications, the availability of counseling and the publication of success rates.

I think the federal government can also insist through its ability to control dollars that flow for reimbursement on standardized and routinized collection of information. It should not be voluntary, it should be mandatory. We shouldn't have to depend upon 41 centers voluntarily telling us what they are up to and how they are doing.

We should insist upon it, we should demand it.

20 NEW CONCEPTIONS AND GOVERNMENT REGULATION

STATE GOVERNMENTS SHOULD REGULATE THE NEW TECHNOLOGIES

George Annas

George Annas is the Edward R. Utley Professor of Health Law at Boston University in Boston, Massachusetts. He teaches in the schools of medicine and public health.

Points to Consider:

1. What are the legal options for regulating the new reproductive technologies?

2. How has the federal government been involved in the past?

3. What role have the states played?

4. Who is the gestational mother and why should she be initially presumed as the legal mother in all surrogate parenting arrangements?

5. Why should regulation be left mainly to the states?

Excerpted from the testimony of George Annas before the House Select Committee on Children, Youth, and Families, May 21, 1987.

Regulation of the new reproductive technologies is primarily a matter for the individual states.

When reviewing the legal options for regulation on both the state and federal level, it will be useful to keep in mind the "pressure points" at which regulation can be brought to bear. In general, these will be: control of medical practice; control of human experimentation; defining the presumptive rearing father and mother; granting legal protection to the extracorporeal human embryo; legal provisions for donor screening and record confidentiality; regulation of commerce in gametes and embryos; and attaching conditions to the delivery of medical services that are paid for by government programs. Protecting the interests of children, for example, will require detailed record-keeping concerning their genetic parents.

Overview of Regulatory Activity to Date

It is fair to say that the federal government has not engaged in any regulatory activity in this area. On the other hand, the federal government has over the last 13 years formed three important commissions that have made recommendations regarding the new reproductive technologies: The National Commission, the Ethics Advisory Board, and the President's Commission on Bioethics; and is in the process of forming another (the Congressional Biomedical Ethics Board).

States have been a bit more active in artificial insemination by donor (AID) [more than half of the states have laws making the husband of the impregnated woman the child's father for all legal purposes so long as he has consented to AID], and a number of states have regulations related to fetal research. But no states have specific statutes on in vitro fertilization (IVF), surrogate embryo transfer (SET) or gamete intrafallopian transfer (GIFT). Since the regulation of medical practice is primarily a state function, regulation of the actual delivery of these technologies is almost always primarily a task for the individual states.

States could also regulate the new reproductive technologies indirectly by statutorily defining which woman, as between a gestational, genetic, and planned-rearing mother would have presumptive rearing rights and obligations with respect to the child. I believe *states should enact statutes that clearly define the gestational mother* (i.e., the woman who gives birth to the child) *as the irrefutably presumed mother for all legal purposes.* This is because of her gestational contribution to the child, and

140

the fact that she will definitely be present at the birth, be easily and certainly identifiable, and available to care for the child. Such a law would have the effect of helping to make legitimate and protect children born from SET, but would give a so-called surrogate mother the right to retain her children even in the face of a prior contractual agreement to give it up for adoption or to relinquish parental rights to the child after birth. She could do either, but only *after* the child was born and the standard waiting period for adoption or relinquishment of parental rights had expired. This presumption would also operate in the case of ovum donation in a manner analogous to AID (sperm donation): the gestational, not the genetic mother, would be the presumptive rearing mother.

Overview of Federal Authority

In the area of health care in general, and the new reproductive technologies in particular, Congress can act in areas where the federal government has indirect authority: primarily taxation and spending, and interstate commerce.

The most important area in which Congress has used its power to spend to adopt regulations related to the new reproductive technologies has been in the area of research on human subjects, and most physicians and institutions engaged in research on these technologies must follow federal requirements for such research.

Regulation of interstate commerce can involve a ban on the sale of an article. Congress has indicated its willingness to ban the purchase and sale of human body parts, and could certainly ban the interstate sale of human embryos (and sperm and ova as well). In 1984, for example, Congress passed the "National Organ Transplant Act." While most of the Act is aimed at promoting organ transplantation in the United States, Title III is directed exclusively toward prohibiting organ purchases. It's operative section reads:

> It shall be unlawful for any person to knowingly acquire, receive, or otherwise transfer any human organ for valuable consideration for use in human transplantation if the transfer affects interstate commerce.

For the purpose of this act, "human organ" is defined to mean "the human kidney, liver, heart, lung, pancreas, bone marrow, cornea, eye, bone, and skin. . ." A violation carries a five year maximum prison sentence, and a $50,000 fine. *Congress should amend this statute to include human embryos among the items it is unlawful to sell.* The purpose would be to protect children by preventing them from being viewed as and treated as commodities. . . .

Constitutional Limits on Regulation

With respect to the new reproductive technologies, we need to examine the underlying values at stake in procreative privacy to delineate the scope of this right. These include self-identity, self-expression, freedom of association, freedom to make decisions that drastically affect one's identity, and rights to have intimate relationships with a view toward producing a child. Although the Supreme Court is badly split on the reach of privacy outside of a heterosexual union, there is no such split concerning privacy within a heterosexual union when that union is aimed at procreation.

All members of the Supreme Court would thus likely conclude that IVF, SET, and GIFT, if conducted within the context of marriage at least (and probably if done in any "stable" heterosexual relationship) are to be viewed as within the ambit of the "right to privacy." Accordingly, only laws similar to those endorsed by the Supreme Court to regulate previable abortions (i.e., those aimed primarily at restricting performance to physicians, monitoring the safety and efficacy of the procedures, and insuring informed consent) could be used to regulate these activities. AID regulations could be stricter, since they involve another participant — the sperm donor — and could include screening rules and procedures as well. Where nonprocreation issues are at stake, or where public participation is sought that might harm others, including the resulting children, banning altogether might be permissible. Examples would include commercial surrogate motherhood, selling human embryos, and experimentation on human embryos. The view of one religion alone (e.g., the Catholic Church) that any or all of these techniques are "illicit" would, in itself, be an insufficient rationale

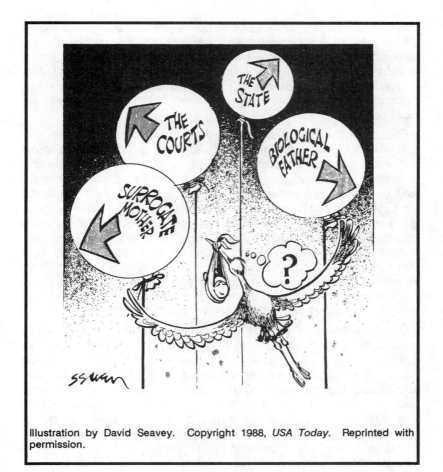

Illustration by David Seavey. Copyright 1988, *USA Today*. Reprinted with permission.

to ban them.

Conclusion

Regulation of the new reproductive technologies is primarily a matter for the individual states. Just as they have regulated adoption, custody, marriage, medical licensing and medical practice, it seems most reasonable for the states to regulate the practice of new reproductive technologies insofar as they are seen as medical procedures and performed by physicians. Regulations in the area of quality control and monitoring, safety, record keeping, inspection and licensing, consent, the identification and obligations of mothers and fathers, and requirements for donor screening, are all well within the traditional state activities and regulation in these areas and would not raise any major social policy implications. In extreme cases, such as banning the sale of human embryos or experimentation with human embryos, statutes would have to be carefully drawn (so as not to be voided for vagueness) and based on a reasonable state policy designed to protect the common good and preventing children from being treated like commodities.

Federal activity in the new reproductive technologies, on the other hand, has been restricted to setting up and financing national commissions and groups of various kinds to study the scientific, legal and ethical issues involved in these practices, and to making recommendations on what actions various private and governmental organizations should take. The federal government could, however, become involved in its own "traditional" areas, such as regulation of interstate commerce, forbidding the sale of human tissue, regulating "false and deceptive" advertising, and promulgating rules for human research, without any major implications. Major federal involvement, however, seems reasonable only when related directly or indirectly to federal financing of these technologies.

Government has only the most limited role in preventing contraception and prohibiting abortion (mainly health and safety of the adult participants), but has a potentially much higher role in the new reproductive technologies: not only protecting the interests of the adults to quality services and informed consent, but also taking reasonable steps to protect the interests of future children that are "created" by these methods. Regulations that are firmly grounded in reasonable steps to protect these children are legitimate, and likely to enjoy broad societal support.

THE FROZEN EMBRYOS

This activity may be used as an individualized study guide for students in libraries and resource centers or as a discussion catalyst in small group and classroom discussions.

DEFINING THE ISSUE

Pretend that a married couple has a dispute in divorce court over their four frozen embryos. These embryos were created in vitro by his sperm and her eggs because of the couple's infertility problems. Previously, doctors had tried unsuccessfully to implant two embryos in the woman's uterus. After the divorce, what should be done with the frozen embryos?

Guidelines (Part A)

Examine the following questions as a guide to individual reflection, class discussion, or small group interaction.

1. What should be done with the frozen embryos?

2. Who should decide the issue?

3. What arguments can be made for giving the embryos to the wife?

4. What arguments can be made for giving them to the husband?

5. What arguments can be made for giving them to a clinic that provides comprehensive services in the area of new reproductive technologies?

6. What arguments can be made for destroying the embryos?

7. What other options can you think of?

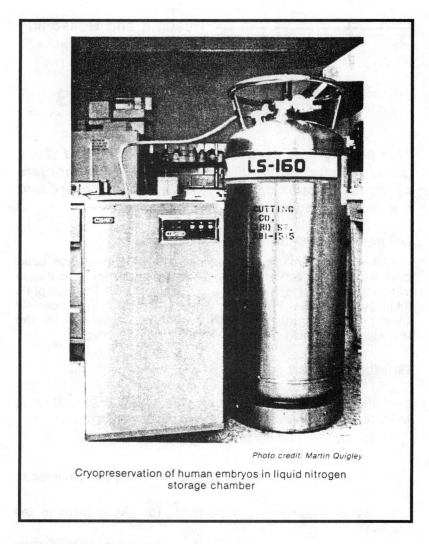

Photo credit: Martin Quigley

Cryopreservation of human embryos in liquid nitrogen storage chamber

Guidelines (Part B)

Evaluate the statements below by using the method indicated.

Place the letter [B] in front of any sentence that is an example of editorial bias or opinion. Place the letter [N] in front of any sentence that is not an example of editorial bias or opinion.

1. A judge should decide the fate of the frozen embryos.

2. The procedure of freezing embryos is immoral and should

be prohibited by law.

3. A special panel of doctors and scholars specializing in medical ethics should decide the fate of the frozen embryos.

4. The wife should decide the fate of the frozen embryos because she went through the most difficult medical procedures.

5. Frozen embryos should be regarded as property in a divorce settlement.

6. Frozen embryos should be regarded as human life from the moment of conception.

7. Frozen embryos have no moral rights and do not have to be treated as human life.

8. All couples by law must be required to say what should be done with their frozen embryos before fertilization takes place should they both die or get a divorce.

9. The frozen embryos should be divided in this case, two for the wife and two for the husband.

10. Whichever spouse pays for the medical procedure should gain custody of the four frozen embryos.

11. The frozen embryos should go to the spouse who intends to use them.

12. The frozen embryos should be destroyed.

13. Frozen embryos should remain frozen until they are used or become unfit for use.

APPENDIX

Glossary of Terms

Artificial insemination (AI): The introduction of sperm into a woman's vagina or uterus by noncoital methods, for the purpose of conception.

Chlamydia: An STD caused by the bacteria *Chlamydia trachomatis*. In women, chlamydial infection accounts for 25 to 50 percent of the pelvic inflammatory disease cases seen each year. Chlamydia is the most common STD in the United States today.

Chromosome: A rod-shaped body in a cell nucleus that carries the genes that convey hereditary characteristics.

Cleavage: The stage of cell division that takes place immediately after fertilization and that lasts until the cells begin to segregate and differentiate and to develop into a blastocyst.

Cryopreservation: The preservation of sperm, embryos, and oocytes by freezing them at extremely low temperatures.

Donor gametes: Eggs or sperm donated by individuals for medically assisted conception.

Ectopic pregnancy: A pregnancy that occurs outside the uterus, usually in a fallopian tube.

Embryo: Term used to describe the stages of growth from the second to the ninth week following conception. During this period cell differentiation proceeds rapidly and the brain, eyes, heart, upper and lower limbs, and other organs are formed.

Embryo donation: The transfer from one woman to another of an embryo obtained by artificial insemination and lavage or, more commonly, by IVF.

Embryo lavage: A flushing of the uterus to recover a preimplantation embryo.

Embryo transfer: The transfer of an in vitro fertilized egg from its laboratory dish into the uterus of a woman.

Extracorporeal embryo: An embryo maintained outside the body.

Fallopian tube: Either of a pair of tubes that conduct the egg from the ovary to the uterus. Fertilization normally occurs within this structure. Blocked or scarred fallopian tubes are a leading source of infertility in women.

Fertilization: The penetration of an oocyte by a sperm and subsequent combining of maternal and paternal DNA.

Fetus: The embryo becomes a fetus after approximately 9 weeks in the uterus. This stage of development lasts from 9 weeks until birth and is marked by the growth and specialization of organ function.

Gamete: A reproductive cell. In a man, the gametes are sperm; in a woman, they are eggs, or ova.

Gamete intrafallopian transfer (GIFT): A technique of medically assisted conception in which mature oocytes are surgically removed from a woman's body and then reintroduced, together with sperm, through a catheter threaded into the fallopian tubes, where it is hoped fertilization will take place.

Gene: The portion of a DNA molecule that consists of an ordered sequence of nucleotide bases and constitutes the basic unit of heredity.

Gonorrhea: An STD caused by the bacteria *Nesseria gonorrheae.* If the infection is not treated in women, it can spread to the uterus and the fallopian tubes, causing pelvic inflammatory disease. In men, it can cause epididymitis and can affect semen quality.

Impotence: The inability to achieve or maintain an erection.

Implantation: The process by which the fertilized oocyte (zygote) becomes attached to the wall of the uterus (endometrium).

In vitro: Literally "in glass"; pertaining to a biological process or reaction taking place in an artificial environment, usually a laboratory.

In vitro fertilization (IVF): A technique of medically assisted conception (sometimes referred to as "test tube" fertilization) in which mature oocytes are removed from a woman's ovary and fertilized with sperm in a laboratory. (See *embryo transfer.*)

In vivo: Literally "in the living"; pertaining to a biological process or reaction taking place in a living cell or organism.

In vivo fertilization: The fertilization of an egg by a sperm within a woman's body. The sperm may be introduced by artificial insemination or by coitus.

Infertility: Inability of a couple to conceive after 12 months of intercourse without contraception.

Intracervical insemination: Artificial insemination technique in which sperm are placed in or near the cervical canal of the female reproductive tract, using a syringe or a catheter, for the purpose of conception.

Intraperitoneal insemination: Artificial insemination technique in which sperm are introduced into the body cavity between the uterus and the rectum, after ovulation has been induced, for the purpose of conception.

Intrauterine device (IUD): Contraceptive device inserted through the cervix into the uterine cavity.

Laparoscopy: Direct visualization of the ovaries and the exterior of the fallopian tubes and uterus by means of a laparoscope (a long, narrow, illuminated instrument) introduced through a small surgical incision below the navel, to evaluate any abnormalities. Surgical procedures may also be performed using this method.

Menstrual cycle: The process of ovulation in which an oocyte matures each month in a follicle produced on the surface of the ovary. At ovulation, the follicle ruptures and the oocyte is released into the body cavity and enters the fallopian tube. If fertilization and implantation do not occur, the uterine lining is sloughed off, producing menstrual flow. The normal menstrual cycle is about 28 days.

Noncoital reproduction: Reproduction other than by sexual intercourse.

Ovaries: Paired female sex glands in which ova are developed and stored and the hormones estrogen and progesterone are produced.

Ovulation: The discharge of an oocyte from a woman's ovary, generally around the midpoint of the menstrual cycle.

Ovum (pl. ova): The female egg or oocyte, formed in an ovary.

Ovum donor: A woman who donates an ovum or ova to another woman.

Prostate gland: Male gland that supplies part of the fluid of the semen.

Semen: A fluid consisting of secretions from the male's seminal vesicles, prostate, and from the glands adjacent to the urethra. Semen carries sperm and is ejaculated during intercourse.

Sexual dysfunction: The inability to achieve normal sexual intercourse for reasons such as impotence, premature ejaculation, and retrograde ejaculation in the man or of vaginismus in the woman.

Sexually transmitted diseases (STDs): Infectious diseases transmitted primarily by sexual contact, including syphilis, gonorrhea, chlamydia, herpes, and acquired immunodeficiency syndrome.

Sperm: The male reproductive cell, or gamete. Normal sperm have symmetrically oval heads, stout midsections, and long tapering tails.

Sperm bank: A place in which sperm are stored by cryopreservation for future use in artificial insemination.

Surrogate gestational mother: A woman who gestates and carries to term an embryo to which she is not genetically related, with the intention of relinquishing the child at birth.

Surrogate mother: A woman who is artifically inseminated and carries an embryo to term, with the intention of relinquishing the child at birth.

Testes: Also known as the testicles, the paired male sex glands in which sperm and the steroid hormone testosterone are produced.

Testosterone: A steroid hormone, or androgen, produced in the testes that affects sperm production and male sex characteristics.

Tubal ligation: The sterilization of a woman by surgical excision of a small section of each fallopian tube.

Ultrasound: The use of high-frequency sound waves focused on the body to obtain a video image of internal tissues, organs, and structures. Ultrasound is particularly useful for in utero examinations of a developing fetus, for evaluation of the development of ovarian follicles, and for the guided retrieval of oocytes for IVF and GIFT.

Uterine lavage: A flushing of the uterus to recover a preimplantation embryo.

Vasectomy: Sterilization of a man by surgical excision of a part of the vas deferens.

Zygote: A fertilized oocyte formed by the fusion of egg and sperm, containing DNA from both.

BIBLIOGRAPHY I

Religious Perspectives

1. Bleich, J.D., *Judaism and Healing* (New York, NY: Katav, 1981).

2. Bush, L., "Ethical Issues in Reproductive Medicine: A Mormon Perspective," *Dialogue: A Journal of Mormon Thought* 18(2):41-66, summer 1985.

3. Commission on Theology and Church Relations, Lutheran Church-Missouri Synod, *Human Sexuality: A Theological Perspective* (St. Louis, MO: Social Concerns Committee, 1981).

4. Creighton, P., *Artificial Insemination by Donor* (Toronto, Ontario: Anglican Book Center, 1977).

5. Division of Theological Studies, Lutheran Council in the U.S., *In Vitro Fertilization* (New York, NY: 1983).

6. Fletcher, J., *Morals and Medicine* (Boston, MA: Bacon Press, 1960).

7. General Conference, Mennonite Church, "Resolution on Sexuality" (adopted in 1985).

8. Harakas, S., *Contemporary Moral Issues Facing the Orthodox Christian* (Minneapolis, MN: Light & Life Publishing Co., 1982).

9. Jones, D.G., *Brave New People* (Leicester, England: Inter Varsity Press, 1984).

10. Lubow, A., Secretary, Law Committee, Rabbinic Assembly, personal communication, May 5, 1987.

11. McCormick, R., *Notes on Moral Theology: 1981-84* (Washington, DC: University Press of America, 1985).

12. National Council of the Churches of Christ in the U.S.A., *Genetic Sciences for Human Benefit* (New York, NY: National Council, 1986).

13. Nelson, J., and Rohricht, J.A.S., *Human Medicine* (Minneapolis, MN: Augsburg Publishing House, 1984).

14. Numbers, R., and Amundsen, R., *Caring and Curing* (New York, NY: Macmillan, 1986).

15. Office of the General Assembly, Presbyterian Church, *The*

Covenant of Life and the Caring Community (New York, NY: Office of the General Assembly, 1983).

16. Provonsha, J., "Surrogate Procreation—An Ethical Dilemma" (Loma Linda, CA: an unpublished lecture made available by the Center for Christian Bioethics, Loma Linda University).

17. Ramsey, P., *Fabricated Man* (New Haven, CT: Yale University Press, 1970).

18. Smith, D., *Health and Medicine in the Anglican Tradition* (New York, NY: Crossroad Publishing Co., 1986).

19. Talbot, N.A., Manager, Committees on Publication, First Church of Christ Scientist, personal communication, March 11, 1987.

20. World Council of Churches, *Faith and Science in an Unjust World,* vol. 2 (Philadelphia, PA: Fortress Press, 1983).

Feminist Views

1. Andrews, L.B., "Feminist Perspectives on Reproductive Technologies," paper presented at *A Forum on Reproductive Law for the 1990's,* New York, NY, May 18, 1987.

2. Arditti, R., Duelli-Klein, R., and Minden, S. (eds.), *Test Tube Women: What Future for Motherhood?* (Boston, MA: Pandora Press, 1984).

3. Choderow, N., *The Reproduction of Mothering* (Berkeley, CA: University of California Press, 1978).

4. Corea, G., *The Hidden Malpractice: How American Medicine Mistreats Women*, 2d ed. (New York, NY: Harper & Row, 1985).

5. Corea, G., *The Mother Machine: Reproductive Technologies from Artificial Insemination to Artificial Wombs* (New York, NY: Harper & Row, 1985).

6. Gallagher, J., "Fetal Personhood and Women's Policy," *Women's Biology and Public Policy,* V. Sapiro (ed.), (Beverly Hills, CA: Sage, 1985).

7. Gilligan, C., *In a Different Voice: Psychological Theory and Women's Development* (Cambridge, MA: Harvard University Press, 1982).

8. Hartsock, N.C.M., *Money Sex, and Power: Toward a Feminist Historical Materialism* (New York, NY: Longman, Inc.,

1983).

9. Holmes, H.B., Hoskins, B., and Gross, M. (eds.), *The Custom Made Child?* (Clifton, NJ: Humana Press, 1981).

10. Hubbard, R., and Sanford, W., "New Reproductive Technologies," *The New Our Bodies, Ourselves*, The Boston Women's Health Book Collective (eds.) (New York, NY: Simon & Schuster, 1984).

11. Jaggar, A.M., *Feminist Politics and Human Nature* (Totowa, NJ: Rowman & Allanheld, 1983).

12. Rich, A., *Of Woman Born* (New York, NY: W.W.Norton & Co., 1977).

13. Rothman, B.K., *In Labor: Women and Power in the Birthplace* (New York, NY: W.W. Norton & Co., 1982).

14. Rothman, B.K., *The Tentative Pregnancy: Prenatal Diagnosis and the Future of Motherhood* (New York, NY: Viking Press, 1986).

15. Rothman, B.K., "Feminism and the New Reproductive Technologies," prepared for the Office of Technology Assessment, U.S. Congress, June 1987.

16. Rothman, B.K., *Recreating Motherhood* (New York, NY: W.W. Norton & Co., in press).

17. Ruzek, S.B., *The Women's Health Movement: Feminist Alternatives to Medical Control* (New York, NY: Praeger Publishers, 1979).

18. Treblicott, J. (ed.), *Mothering: Essays in Feminist Theory* (Totowa, N.J.: Rowman & Allanheld, 1983).

19. Wikler, N., "Society's Response to the New Reproductive Technologies: The Feminist Perspectives," *Southern California Law Review* 59:1043-1057, 1986.

Ethical Considerations

1. American College of Obstetricians and Gynecologists, *Ethical Issues in Human In Vitro Fertilization and Embryo Placement* (Washington, DC: 1986).

2. American Fertility Society, Ethics Committee, "Ethical Considerations of the New Reproductive Technologies," *Fertility and Sterility* 46:1S-94S, 1986.

3. American Hospital Association, "Statement on a Patient's Bill of Rights," *Hospitals* 47:41, 1973.

4. American Medical Association, Judicial Council, *Opinions and Reports* (Chicago, IL: 1968).

5. Blackwell, R.E., Carr, B.R., Chang, R.J., et al., "Are We Exploiting the Infertile Couple?" *Fertility and Sterility* 48:735-739, 1987.

6. Brody, B.A., "Religious and Secular Perspectives About Infertility Prevention and Treatment," prepared for the Office of Technology Assessment, U.S. Congress, Washington, DC, June 1987.

7. Caplan, A.L., "The New Technologies in Reproduction—New Ethical Problems," *Annals of the New York Academy of Sciences,* in press, 1988.

8. Congregation for the Doctrine of the Faith, *Instruction on Respect for Human Life in Its Origin and on the Dignity of Procreation* (Vatican City: 1987).

9. Daniels, N., "Am I My Parents' Keeper?" *Midwest Studies in Philosophy* 7:517-520, 1982.

10. Dickens, B.M., Faculty of Law, University of Toronto, Toronto, Canada, personal communication, Aug. 28, 1987.

11. Dionne, E.J., "Paris Widow Wins Suit to Use Sperm; Court Decides Against Sperm Bank in Plea from Wife of Man Who Died in 1983," *New York Times,* Aug. 2, 1984.

12. Edelstein, L., "The Hippocratic Oath: Text, Translation and Interpretation," *Ancient Medicine: Selected Papers of Ludwig Edelstein,* O. Tempkin and C. Tempkin (eds.) (Baltimore, MD: Johns Hopkins University Press, 1967).

13. Engelhardt, H.T., Jr., Center for Ethics, Medicine and Public Issues, Baylor College of Medicine, Houston, TX, personal communication, June 24, 1987.

14. Flower, M.J., "The Neuromaturation of the Fetus," *Journal of Medicine and Philosophy* 10:237-251, 1985.

15. Fried, C., *Right and Wrong* (Cambridge, MA: Harvard University Press, 1978).

16. Hart, H.L.A., "Are There Any Natural Rights?" *Rights*, D. Lyons (ed.) (Belmont, CA: Wadsworth Publishing Co., 1979).

17. Hegel, G.W.F., *The Philosophy of Right*, Trans. T.M. Knox (Oxford, UK: Clarendon Press, 1952).

18. Jansen, R., "Ethics in Infertility Treatment," *The Infertile Couple,* R. Pepperell, C. Wood, and B. Hudson (eds.) (New York, NY: Churchill Livingstone, in press).

19. Jones, H.W., and Schrader, C., "The Process of Human

Fertilization: Implications for Moral Status," *Fertility and Sterility* 48:189-192, 1987.

20. Kuhse, H., and Singer, P., "The Moral Status of the Embryo," *Test-Tube Babies,* W. Walters and P. Singer (eds.) (Melbourne, Australia: Oxford University Press, 1982).

21. Mann, D., "Growth Means Doom," *Science Digest* 4:79-81, 1983.

22. McCormick, R.A., "Reproductive Technologies: Ethical Issues," *Encyclopedia of Bioethics*, W.T. Reich (ed.) (New York, NY: Macmillan/Free Press, 1978).

23. McCormick, R.A., "Vatican Asks Governments to Curb Birth Technology and to Outlaw Surrogates," *New York Times*, March 11, 1987.

24. Mill, J.S., *Utilitarianism and Other Writings* (New York, NY: The New American Library, Inc., 1962).

25. Moraczewski, A.S., Regional Director, Pope John XXIII Medical-Moral Research and Education Center, Houston, TX, personal communication, August 28, 1987.

26. Nielsen, K., "Radical Egalitarian Justice: Justice as Equality," *Social Theory and Practice* 5:209-226, 1979.

27. Nozick, R., *Anarchy, State and Utopia* (New York, NY: Basic Books, 1974).

28. President's Commission for the Study of Ethical Problems in Medicine and Biomedical and Behavioral Research, *Securing Access to Health Care* (Washington, DC: U.S. Government Printing Office, 1983).

29. Rawls, J., *A Theory of Justice* (Cambridge, MA: Belknap Press of Harvard University Press, 1971).

30. Robertson, J.A., "Embryos, Families and Procreative Liberty: The Legal Structure of the New Reproduction," *Southern California Law Review* 59:971-987, 1986.

31. Robertson, J.A., "Ethical and Legal Issues in Cryopreservation of Human Embryos," *Fertility and Sterility* 47:371-381, 1987.

32. Sacred Congregation for the Doctrine of the Faith, *Declaration on Procured Abortion* 66:12-13, 1974.

33. Tauer, C.A., "Personhood and Human Embryos and Fetuses," *Journal of Medicine and Philosophy* 10: 253-266, 1985.

34. Thomasma, D.C., Director, Medical Humanities Program, Loyola University Stritch School of Medicine, Chicago, IL, personal communication, March 16, 1987.

35. U.S. Department of Health, Education, and Welfare, Ethics Advisory Board, *HEW Support of Research Involving Human In Vitro Fertilization and Embryo Transfer,* May 4, 1979.

36. Veatch, R.M., *A Theory of Medical Ethics* (New York, NY: Basic Books, 1981).

37. Walters, L., "Ethical Aspects of Medical Confidentiality," *Contemporary Issues in Bioethics,* T. Beauchamp and L. Walters (eds.) (Belmont, CA: Wadsworth Publishing Co., 1982).

BIBLIOGRAPHY II
(ANNOTATED)

Surrogate Mothers

"After Baby M, Motherhood Is Not for Sale: Surrogate Births."
U.S. News & World Report, v. 104, February 15, 1988: 11-12.

The New Jersey Supreme Court decision gave final custody of "Baby M" to her father William Stern, while granting surrogate mother Mary Beth Whitehead visitation rights. Reports the Chief Justice's conclusion that the payment of money to a surrogate mother is "illegal, perhaps criminal, and potentially degrading to women."

Andrade, Jane Carroll. "The Law and Surrogate Motherhood."
State Legislatures, v. 13, July 1987: 24-26.

"The Baby M case has spawned a national debate on the moral and legal aspects of surrogate motherhood. Opinions are personal, and they don't fit neatly into the traditional philosophies of political parties or special interest groups. Now, lawmakers must decide how to deal with the complexities of the issue."

Andrews, Lori B. "The Aftermath of Baby M: Proposed State Laws on Surrogate Motherhood." *Hastings Center Report,* v. 17, Oct.-Nov. 1987: 31-40. LRS87-10421

Describes laws State legislatures are considering on the issue of surrogate motherhood. "Like artificial insemination of the 1950s and 1960s, this new reproductive technology is evoking legislative responses ranging from horrified prohibition to cautious facilitation."

Arditti, Rita. "The Surrogacy Business." *Social Policy*, v. 18, fall 1987: 42-46. LRS87-12402

"The commercialization of women's procreative power promotes the exploitation of women and constitutes an attack on the dignity of all human beings."

Brahams, Diana. "The Hasty British Ban on Commercial Surrogacy." *Hastings Center Report*, v. 17, Feb. 1987: 16-19.

Great Britain's Surrogacy Arrangements Act of 1985 made it a criminal offense for third parties to benefit from surrogacy while leaving voluntary surrogacy lawful.

Donovan, Patricia. "New Reproductive Technologies: Some Legal Dilemmas." *Family Planning Perspectives,* v. 18, Mar.-Apr. 1986: 57-60.

Examines the need for developing a legal framework to regulate the use of alternative reproductive technologies, such as surrogate motherhood.

Kruse, Richard A. "The Strange Case of Baby M." *Human Life Review,* v. 13, fall 1987: 27-34. LRS87-12396

Charges that the Bergen County (N.J.) Superior Court Judge Harvey R. Sorkow's 1987 decision in the "Baby M" surrogate case "omitted any consideration of the ethical, philosophical, or public-policy aspects of the problem." Contends that "contracts and commercialism should never enter into" the decision to have and to raise a child.

Lacayo, Richard. "Whose Child Is This? Baby M. and the Agonizing Dilemma of Surrogate Motherhood." *Time*, v. 129, Jan. 19, 1987: 56-58.

Looks at selected elements of the legal case to be decided by the New Jersey Superior Court. Reviews ethical arguments for and against surrogacy.

O'Brien, Shari. "The Itinerant Embryo and the Neo-nativity Scene: Bifurcating Biological Maternity" *Utah Law Review*, v. 1987, no. 1, 1987: 1-33. LRS87-5611

"This article highlights the legal and socio-ethical implications of surrogate embryo transfer and surrogate gestation, a pair of distinct, recently developed reproductive technologies that fragment biological maternity."

Pollitt, Katha. "Contracts and Apple Pie: The Strange Case of Baby M." *Nation*, v. 244, May 23, 1987: 667, 682-686, 688.

Examines the Baby M trial as a means of looking at the legality of surrogate motherhood.